Fit for Duty

Robert Hoffman, MS
Human Kinetics

Thomas R. Collingwood, PhD
Fitness Intervention Technologies

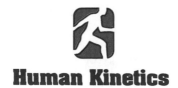

Human Kinetics

Library of Congress Cataloging-in-Publication Data

Hoffman, Robert, 1947-
    Fit for duty / Robert Hoffman, Thomas R. Collingwood.
       p.   cm.
    Includes bibliographical references and index.
    ISBN 0-87322-877-4 (pbk.)
  1. Police--Health and hygiene.   2. Physical fitness.
  I. Collingwood, Thomas R.   II. Title.
  HV7936.H4H627   1995
  613' .0243632--dc20   94-44690
                                                CIP

ISBN: 0-87322-877-4

Developmental Editors: Lori Garrett and Julia Anderson; **Assistant Editor:** Jacqueline Blakley; **Copyeditor:** Robert Chapdu; **Proofreader:** Dena Popara; **Indexer:** Theresa J. Schaefer; **Text Design and Layout:** Doug Burnett; **Cover Designer:** Keith Blomberg; **Photographer:** Will Zehr; **Illustrator:** Tim Offenstein; **Printer:** United Graphics

Human Kinetics books are available at special discounts for bulk purchase. Special editions or book excerpts can also be created to specification. For details, contact the Special Sales Manager at Human Kinetics.

Printed in the United States of America   10 9

Human Kinetics
Web site: www.HumanKinetics.com

United States: Human Kinetics, P.O. Box 5076, Champaign, IL 61825-5076
800-747-4457
e-mail: humank@hkusa.com

Canada: Human Kinetics, 475 Devonshire Road, Unit 100, Windsor, ON N8Y 2L5
800-465-7301 (in Canada only)
e-mail: orders@hkcanada.com

Europe: Human Kinetics, 107 Bradford Road, Stanningley
Leeds LS28 6AT, United Kingdom
+44 (0) 113 255 5665
e-mail: hk@hkeurope.com

Australia: Human Kinetics, 57A Price Avenue, Lower Mitcham, South Australia 5062
08 8277 1555
e-mail: liahka@senet.com.au

New Zealand: Human Kinetics, P.O. Box 105-231, Auckland Central
09-523-3462
e-mail: hkp@ihug.co.nz

Contents

Preface   vii

Acknowledgments   ix

Introduction   xi

PART I   FIT FOR DUTY, FIT FOR LIFE   1

Chapter 1   What Fitness Means to You   3

What Is Fitness?   3

Fitness on the Job   5

Americans' Fitness and Health   6

Officers' Fitness   8

Officers' Health   8

Benefits of a Fitness Program   9

Chapter 2   How Fit Are You?   11

Screening Before Testing   11

Agency Fitness Testing   13

Assessing Your Fitness Level   13

PART II   PHYSICAL FITNESS   21

Chapter 3   Principles of Exercise   23

Principle #1: Individuality   23

Principle #2: Adaptation   24

Principle #3: Overload   24

Principle #4: Progression   24

Principle #5: Specificity   24

Principle #6: Regularity   25

Principle #7: Recovery   25

Principle #8: Balance   26

Principle #9: Variety   26

Principle #10: Reversibility   26

Principle #11: Moderation   27

FITT   27

Chapter 4   Cardiovascular Endurance   29

   What Is Cardiovascular Endurance?   30

   Designing Your Program   30

   Environmental Guidelines   34

   Suggested Readings   36

**Chapter 5   Resistance Training for Muscular Strength
and Endurance**   37

   What Are Muscular Strength and Muscular Endurance?   37

   Designing Your Program   39

   Additional Strength Training Tips   44

   Suggested Readings   48

Chapter 6   Flexibility   49

   What Is Flexibility?   49

   Designing Your Program   50

   Additional Flexibility Training Tips   53

   Warm-Up and Cool-Down   53

   Suggested Readings   54

Chapter 7   Anaerobic Fitness   55

   What Is Anaerobic Fitness?   55

   Designing Your Program   56

   Developing the Anaerobic Training Plan   57

   Additional Training Tips   58

   Suggested Reading   58

PART III   LIFESTYLE COMPONENTS OF FITNESS   59

Chapter 8   Diet and Nutrition   61

   What Is Nutrition?   61

   Classes of Nutrients   61

   Basic Nutritional Goals   65

   Suggested Readings   67

Chapter 9   Weight Management   69

   What Is Weight Management?   69

   Why Is Weight Management Important?   70

   Principles of Losing Weight   70

   Developing a Weight Management Plan   71

   Tips for Changing Eating Behaviors   72

   Suggested Readings   73

Chapter 10 Stress Management   75

   What Is Stress?   75

   Avoidable and Unavoidable Stressors   77

   Relaxation Techniques   78

   Additional Tips for Reducing Stress   78

   Suggested Readings   79

Chapter 11 Smoking Cessation   81

   What's So Bad About Cigarettes?   82

   Effects of Second-Hand Smoke   82

   Benefits of Quitting   83

   How Do You Quit?   83

   Suggested Readings   85

Chapter 12 Substance Abuse Prevention   87

   Areas of Concern Regarding Substance Abuse   88

   Alcohol   88

   Drugs   89

   Steroids   90

   Suggested Readings   91

PART IV   SETTING COURSE AND STAYING WITH IT   93

Chapter 13 Goal Setting   95

   Developing Goals   95

   Determining Your Fitness Goals   97

   Filling Out the Goal-Setting Worksheet   101

Chapter 14 Realistic Expectations   103

   What Is the Extent of the Problem?   104

   Predictors of Exercise Program Quitters   104

   Dangerous Times   104

   Dropping Out   105

   How to Avoid Slippage Problems   106

   Ways to Improve Your Own Perseverance   107

   Making a Contract   108

   Suggested Readings   108

Appendix A   Weight Training Exercises   111

Appendix B   Static Stretching Exercises   115

Appendix C   Professional Support Organizations   123

Index   125

About the Authors   131

Preface

Why are you reading this book? We hope it's because you have decided to improve your level of fitness, and recognize that this book is aimed directly at you, the law enforcement officer. Any officer who wants to improve his or her job performance, health, and quality of life will benefit from this book.

This handbook is a fitness reference for all law enforcement officers, regardless of fitness ability. While it can be used by officers to develop their individual programs, it can also be used to complement instruction or training presented as part of the *FitForce* program. *FitForce* is a multi-level program which provides training for officers to become fitness coordinators and instructors; ongoing education in the form of Fitness Kits, which include videos, newsletters, and other printed materials; and a consultation service for agencies subscribing to the Fitness Kits.

This handbook promotes a total fitness approach, presenting information not only about physical fitness but also about diet and nutrition, weight management, smoking cessation, substance abuse prevention, and stress management. The emphasis is on developing your physical fitness to improve your job performance and your health, and to enhance your enjoyment of leisure time. To accomplish this you will learn how to develop a training plan for each component of physical fitness. The approach for the lifestyle components of total fitness is to alert you to possible problems and direct you to sources of help.

Although the principles of fitness are the same for everyone, this book looks at each element of a fitness program from a law enforcement point of view. It is founded on 20 years of law enforcement fitness experience, as well as feedback from various law enforcement officers from around the country. The principles have been repeatedly tried in the field and found to produce the desired results.

This doesn't mean that what you learn about fitness is specific only to law enforcement officers. The lessons you learn here can be shared with your family and friends. You'll be doing them a favor while you help yourself.

To get the most out of this book, you must interact with it. The book contains examples and some exercises to complete. Some of you may be doing these exercises under the direction of a Fitness Coordinator; others of you will be participating on your own. This book is designed to help you succeed either way.

This book also will help you design your own individualized exercise program. You'll learn how to assess your current fitness level so you'll know where to begin, then set your goals for maintenance or improvement. You can use this book to develop a program that will challenge you, whether you are already fit or just a beginner.

Most important, this book goes beyond merely telling you what to do; it tells you how and why. By reading this book you will increase your fitness knowledge as well as improve your fitness and health.

Part I of the handbook sets the stage for the rest of the book. Chapter 1 shows why fitness is important to law enforcement officers, and chapter 2 allows you to assess your own fitness.

Part II explains physical fitness. It describes the components of physical fitness: how to design a program and how to set goals and evaluate progress. The chapters cover the principles of exercise, cardiovascular endurance conditioning, muscular strength and endurance conditioning, flexibility, and anaerobic fitness.

Part III discusses the lifestyle components of fitness. This part teaches you how these affect your health as well as your job performance and where to go for additional help. It includes chapters on nutrition, weight management, stress management, smoking cessation, and substance abuse prevention.

Throughout the book, examples based on fictional characters demonstrate each step of the process. Although it is unlikely that your situation will exactly match that of any of these characters, you will learn the process, and that is one key to making the lifestyle

changes necessary to improve performance and health.

The other key to improving health and performance is behavioral change. The process of changing behavior is not hard to understand, but can be difficult to implement. This book will teach you how to make the necessary changes. It will teach how to assess your current fitness level, educate you about training plans, and show you how to set goals.

By reading this far, you have indicated a desire to improve your fitness. The cost to you is a little time. The payoff is substantial. In addition to the benefits noted above, you will look better, feel better about yourself, reduce the stress in your life, and live longer. You are on the right path. You have taken the first step by opening this book. Go for it!

Acknowledgments

We are indebted to many people for helping to publish this book. Obviously, it couldn't have been done without the loyal efforts of the editorial and production staffs of Human Kinetics. In particular, we would like to thank Patricia Sammann, who has become quite an expert in law enforcement fitness, for her review of the manuscript. We would also like to thank Jay Smith, Director of Physical Fitness and Health Maintenance Programs, Massachusetts Criminal Justice Training Council; and John Gnagey, Deputy Chief of the Champaign (IL) Police Department, for their reviews and valuable feedback.

Introduction

Officer Tony Hernandez is a 40-year-old patrolman who has been on the force for 15 years. During that time he has seen his share of street action, but he has also seen more than his share of donut shops and fast-food stands. Two recent events have given Tony serious concerns. The first was receiving the results of his physical exam. The doctor told him that he was 60 pounds overweight and that his body fat was 33% of his total weight. The doctor was concerned about his health, and his wife was worried sick, but Tony was only marginally upset. That is, until the following Tuesday. He and his partner responded to a domestic disturbance call, allegedly involving a gun. As they were racing up to the sixth floor, Tony ran out of gas at the second floor. His partner had to go on without him. A terrible picture flashed in Tony's mind, and when it turned out no gun was involved, he was only mildly relieved. While his partner never said anything to him, the look he gave Tony after the incident spoke volumes. Tony anguished about it. He knew that he couldn't get into shape overnight, but he made a vow that he would make progress and never put his partner in a jam like that again. His agency has a fitness program which consists of mandatory testing but voluntary participation. Up to this point, Tony had chosen to be a nonparticipant. On Wednesday he promised his partner that he was going to change his ways, and to do something about it.

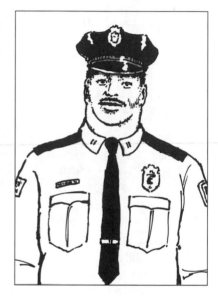

Roosevelt Johnson is a 45-year-old investigator in a sheriff's office. A heavy smoker, Rosie, as he is known to his friends, has high blood pressure and frequent chest pains. In spite of rarely exercising, Rosie is not overweight, and his high school friends kid him about still being the same size as he was during his days as a basketball and football star. Rosie also had two recent experiences which shook him up a bit. While making an arrest, he was involved in a use-of-force situation that really wore him out. It took him far longer to cuff the suspect than it should have, and he was huffing and puffing so much at the end that the suspect was making fun of him. Shortly after this event, his 14-year-old son asked him to play basketball. Within 5 minutes he was too exhausted to continue. Thinking about his approaching retirement, Rosie was frightened about being too unhealthy to enjoy it, or worse yet, dying before he saw his family grow up. Even though his agency did not have a fitness program, he knew that he had to do something about it.

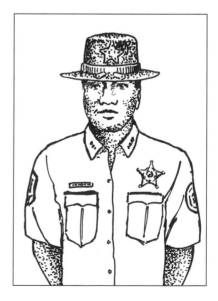

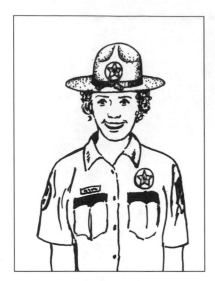

Monique Roberts is a 30-year-old state trooper. Slim and fit looking, Monique is an avid jogger who often enters local road races. In fact, since moving into a new age group, she often places in the top three of the 30- to 34-year-olds. She has a personal goal of becoming the first female member of the state's Special Weapons and Tactics Team. But a recent event has given her a new concern. Arriving at the scene of a traffic accident, Monique did not have enough strength to pull the victim out of the car by herself. Fortunately, another officer happened by and gave her assistance. When the medical personnel arrived, the second officer left to respond to another call. For the second time in twenty minutes Monique learned that the endurance and stamina that she had developed through running wouldn't always be enough—she couldn't push the damaged car onto the shoulder of the road. She then realized that if she was to have any chance of qualifying for SWAT training, she would have to do something about it.

So what did these officers "do about it"? Officers Hernandez and Johnson started fitness programs, and Officer Roberts added a new dimension to her existing program. And by applying the lessons that this book will teach you, they were able to make improvements which had positive effects on their job performance and their personal lives. You'll follow them through the book and use their experiences as examples of each of the learning steps. These officers are fictional, created as composites of real-life officers who are in the field today. But the procedures they put to use have been tried and found successful.

Still not convinced about the need for fitness for law enforcement officers? Then please read Part I.

PART I

Fit for Duty, Fit for Life

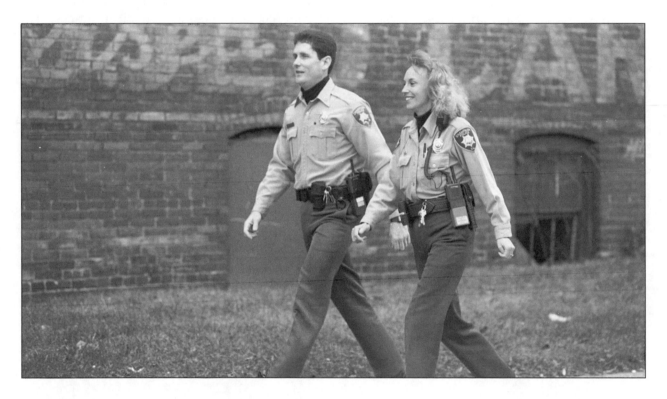

Every day, there is some item in the news related to health or fitness. Often the news reports the results of recent research. Health and fitness are newsworthy because people are thirsty for information about them. The public is much more aware of and concerned with health and fitness than ever before. While occasionally the new information conflicts with earlier reports, the research is clear on one point: lifestyle choices that people make every day have a significant bearing on their performance and health.

This increased concern with health and fitness has been equally evident within law enforcement agencies. Visionary administrators as well as police on the beat have come to realize that an officer who is fit will perform better, be healthier, and cost the agency less money in sick time, disability, and liability. The fact that you are reading this book probably means that either you have come to this realization yourself or your agency has provided an opportunity to improve your fitness with a program. In either case, the first part of this book is important to your overall understanding of the issue.

The purpose of Part I is to give you general information about fitness. It will take you from the big picture—how fit America is—to a more specific concern—how fit you are. In between you'll see how fit law enforcement officers are compared to the rest of the population.

Chapter 1 defines total fitness and its components. It discusses why fitness is important to law enforcement officers and gives you some examples of the types of activities that require fitness. You'll read some alarming statistics about the fitness and health of Americans and recognize that these problems aren't caused by germs or viruses but rather by lifestyle choices.

Next, you'll learn about the fitness and health of your fellow officers. You might be surprised to see how you compare to the pub-lic at large. You'll also get a feel for what some law enforcement professional groups have to say about the issue.

Finally, chapter 1 will present the bene-fits of a fitness program. These benefits include improved performance and better health, and they help the organization as well as the individual.

Chapter 2 gives you the opportunity to assess your own fitness level. If your agency does not administer a fitness test, here is a simple test which will give you an idea of your current level of physical fitness. The chapter also gives some precautions to take before beginning an exercise program.

CHAPTER 1

What Fitness Means to You

As you read through this chapter, you will progressively add to your fitness knowledge. First you'll learn what fitness is and see some reasons why fitness is important to you. Next you'll learn about the general fitness status of Americans, and more specifically how law enforcement officers compare. Finally, you'll learn the benefits of a fitness program.

What Is Fitness?

You hear the word "fitness" used often, and while you may have an idea of what it means, people use it to describe a number of different conditions and concepts. Generally, when people hear the term they think of physical fitness. Physical fitness is the ability to perform physical activities, such as job tasks, with enough reserve for emergency situations and to enjoy recreational pursuits. While that is an important part of "fitness," there is more

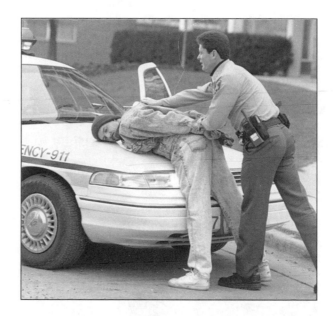

to being fit than just exercise. This handbook is based on a concept of "total fitness." Total fitness is the ability to perform physical activities while being free of health problems. It incorporates the fitness lifestyle areas of nutrition, weight management, stress management, smoking cessation, and substance abuse prevention, along with exercise, to produce maximum performance and health.

Both your health and your performance are affected by your lifestyle. For example, eating correctly will lower your chances for heart diseases and other health problems while providing the energy you need to pursue suspects and engage in use-of-force situations.

This book will concentrate on physical fitness and will help you develop an individual exercise plan to either improve or maintain

---

When you finish this chapter, you will be able to:

- ✪ Know what fitness is.
- ✪ Understand why fitness is important to law enforcement officers.
- ✪ See the fitness status of Americans in general and of law enforcement personnel in particular.
- ✪ Recognize the benefits of a healthy lifestyle.

your current level of physical fitness. Since the other components of total fitness interrelate with physical fitness and each other, you will learn the basics of each component and where to go if you need additional help. If your agency subscribes to the *FitForce* program, the educational component of that program includes Fitness Kits, which will be a source of further information about these important fitness lifestyles.

Before we begin a discussion of the importance of fitness to law enforcement officers, it will help if you understand what comprises physical fitness. As you will learn in more detail in Part II of this book, there are six components of physical fitness:

■ **Cardiovascular endurance (CVE).** This means your ability to perform activity that requires the body to combine its energy sources with oxygen. You may also see it referred to as aerobic power, endurance, stamina, and cardiorespiratory endurance. It is important to law enforcement officers for activities requiring extended effort, such as pursuits of over 2 minutes and use-of-force situations.

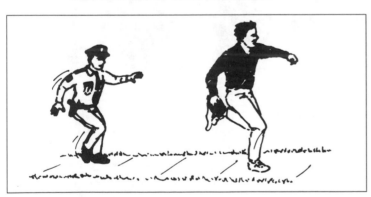

■ **Muscular strength.** This relates to the muscles' ability to generate maximum force. You may also see it referred to as absolute strength. It is important for activities such as pushing a disabled car out of traffic and lifting people or things.

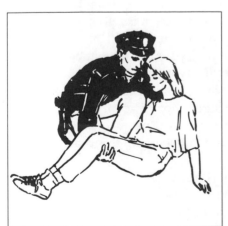

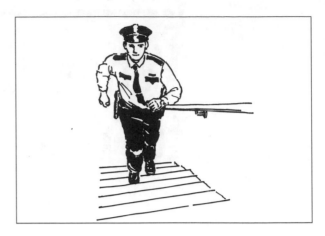

■ **Muscular endurance.** This measures the muscles' capacity to make repeated contractions without too much fatigue. You may also see it referred to as dynamic strength. It is important in use-of-force situations and many other law enforcement scenarios.

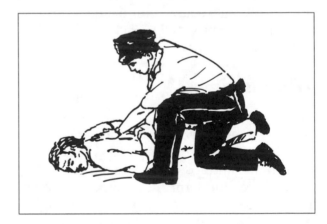

■ **Anaerobic power.** This is the ability to make short, intense bursts of maximal effort. It is important in pursuit situations and other situations requiring short, intense efforts.

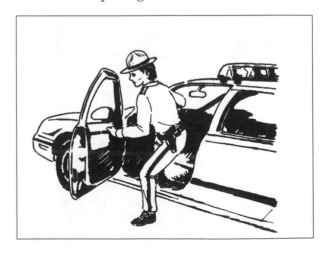

- **Flexibility.** This is the range of motion of part of the body around a joint. It is important for any activities involving bending and reaching.

- **Body composition.** This is the balance between fat and lean tissue in your body.

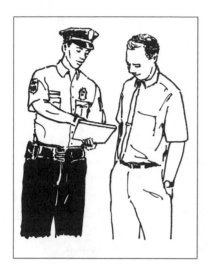

Generally, the lower your percent body fat, the more efficient your movement. An appropriate level of body fat also contributes to good appearance, which can enhance your professional image.

Fitness on the Job

Fitness is important to everyone. The more fit you are, the easier it is to deal with just about every aspect of life. And if being fit can have a positive impact on your home life, just imagine what it can do for your performance on the job!

As you already know, the physical demands of your job may be infrequent but they can be tough. In a pursuit situation, you may be running, climbing, jumping, or using force. To help protect civilians in an emergency, you may have to lift, carry, drag, pull, or push objects. And to make things even more difficult, it's likely that you'll have to go from relative inactivity to high gear with little or no warning. To give you a feeling for the level of effort these tasks entail, here are the results of a survey from the Multijurisdictional Law Enforcement Physical Skills Survey (Wollack & Associates, 1992) that describe some of the demands on law enforcement officers:

- **Running.** The most frequent running tasks lasted less than a minute. However, over 11% of running tasks took over 2 minutes.

Surmounting and avoiding obstacles were required in most running situations.

- **Climbing.** Most fences climbed were 5 feet high or lower. For stairs, one or two flights were usually involved. Quickness was important for both types of climbing.

- **Jumping.** Vaulting and jumping were generally done over obstacles of 3 feet or less.

- **Lifting and carrying.** The majority of lifting and carrying tasks were unassisted, with weights of 50 pounds or less for distances of 20 feet or less.

- **Dragging.** Dragging and pulling tasks were predominantly unassisted, with most objects weighing less than 100 pounds and being moved less than 10 feet.

- **Pushing.** Most of the pushed objects weighed less than 100 pounds and were pushed a distance of less than 10 feet. For vehicles that were pushed, the distance moved was usually more than 30 feet and the move was done in less than a minute.

- **Use of force.** For over 75% of the apprehensions, the amount of resistance was moderate or strong. In the majority of the occurrences, immediate officer attention was required. The time it took to subdue a suspect was equally distributed among 30, 60 and 120 seconds or more.

- **Energy cost.** For many of the sustained physical tasks lasting over 2 minutes (such as pursuits and use-of-force situations) the level of stamina required of officers was often 75%-90% of their maximum capability.

Performing Essential Tasks

You may feel that your job doesn't require you to perform physically exerting tasks often, and so physical fitness isn't crucial. However, you also have to look at the importance of the situations in which fitness is a factor. Many of the physical tasks associated with your job, even if not performed often, can have unfavorable results if failed. Take a look at some of the studies of the frequency and significance of physical tasks in law enforcement.

One study considered the frequency with which each of 20 physical tasks was performed annually, both in absolute numbers and as percentages of work days in a year. The percentages ranged from 1% to 32%, so you might think that the tasks weren't performed often enough to worry about. However, according to Wollack and Associates (1992), inadequate performance of these tasks could have resulted in

- failure to provide needed service (77%-91% of occurrences),

- property loss or damage (28%-55% of occurrences),

- failure to apprehend suspect (32%-85% of occurrences), or

- possible loss of life/injury risk (46%-79% of occurrences).

These results indicate that even low-frequency physical tasks must be performed well when required or the results will be undesirable.

Another study looked at 24 physical tasks to determine their criticality, that is, how serious the consequences may be if a task can't be performed. While only six of the tasks were performed frequently, all 24 were deemed to be critical tasks.

The bottom line is that it doesn't matter how infrequently you may be called on to perform a physical task if it is critical. If you're not fit enough, at best you've failed in your duty; at worst, it may kill you or someone else. It's like the need to maintain firearm skills. You may rarely use your weapon, but when shooting skill is needed, it's critical that you have it.

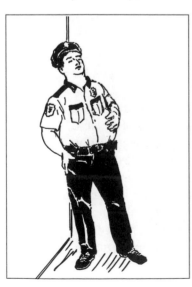

Maintaining a Professional Image

Part of an officer's effectiveness is based on the image he or she presents. A quote from an article in the April 1994 issue of *Law and Order* magazine states: "An officer's image has a direct impact on his or her effectiveness within the community." The public judges officers by their physical appearance and their lifestyles, both of which are tied to fitness.

Fitness as a means to improve officers' images also fits into the recent trend to improve the professionalism of law enforcement officials. Just as that trend has focused on areas such as officers' ethics, cognitive functioning, and interpersonal and social skills, it also should include fitness.

It should be clear by now that an officer's fitness relates to job performance. That's half of the total fitness definition—the capability to perform physical tasks. The other half is officers' health. To get the big picture, let's start with Americans' fitness and health in general, then see how law enforcement officers fare in comparison to the general population.

Americans' Fitness and Health

Americans in general are not as fit as they should be. The consequences of this can mean more than poor job performance—they can lead to disability or death. If that seems overly dramatic, consider these statistics:

- In 1992, cardiovascular (heart) diseases killed more than 900,000 Americans. This rate is half of what it was in 1967, due to smoking cessation, lower cholesterol, and better medical care.

- In 1993, an estimated 526,000 Americans died of cancer, about 1,400 a day. One out of every five deaths in the U.S. is from cancer.

- About 85% of cases of lung cancer are caused by smoking.

- In 1986, Pacific Life Mutual estimated the illness cost of poor nutrition to be $30 million annually.

- Americans have an 8-in-10 chance of experiencing back pain some time in their adult lives.

- About 62 million Americans are being treated for high blood pressure.

- About two thirds of Americans' visits to primary-care physicians are stress related, 112 million people take medication for stress, and industry loses more than $150 billion annually to stress-related problems.

- In 1990, the cost of alcohol-abuse problems was estimated at $70 billion, and the cost of drug abuse at $44 billion.

- In 1990, more than 300,000 Americans took anabolic steroids, and it is estimated that Americans spend $500 million annually on anabolic steroids.

These conditions are not communicable illnesses from viruses or bacteria; they are conditions related to poor fitness. Choices you make about your lifestyle affect these conditions. How you eat, whether you exercise, what stresses you're under, and many more factors in your daily life influence whether you develop them. The good news about these medical problems is that you can do something to combat them. Many of the causes of death and disability are well documented— sedentary living, poor nutrition, obesity, stress, tobacco smoking, and substance abuse.

Sedentary Living

Only 22% of American adults get at least 30 minutes of light to moderate exercise five or more times a week, and less than 10% exercise vigorously three times a week. Studies have shown that sedentary people run twice the risk of coronary heart disease that active people do. They also have a higher rate of stroke and of colon cancer, and may be more prone to back injury and stress-related problems.

Poor Nutrition

Dietary fat currently makes up 34% of the calories in the average American diet. Yet too much dietary fat can create a higher risk of heart disease, breast and colon cancer, and possibly gallbladder disease. Too little fiber can create a risk of colon cancer or diverticulosis; too little calcium can lead to osteoporosis and may relate to colon cancer and high blood pressure.

Obesity

About one third of American adults are overweight. Many are also obese; that is, they have unhealthy amounts of body fat. Obesity has been linked with many chronic diseases such as diabetes, hypertension, and cancer. It also may make orthopedic and lower-back problems worse.

Stress

We all have stress in our lives, but the ability to control stress impacts our health and fitness. Stress can be a secondary risk factor in major health problems such as heart disease, hypertension, cancer, ulcers, and lower-back pain.

Smoking

More than 50 million Americans smoke. Tobacco smoking doubles the chance of heart attacks, causes 20% of the deaths from stroke and 85% of lung cancer, and is linked to other types of cancer, emphysema, and chronic bronchitis. Recent research seems to indicate that second-hand smoke causes health problems for nonsmokers—some studies even estimate that second-hand smoke leads to 47,000 deaths per year. There is also a not-yet-explained connection between smoking and lower-back pain. Despite some recent reduction in the number of smokers, smoking is still responsible for one of every six deaths in the U.S., about 400,000 annually.

Substance Abuse

About 18 million Americans currently have problems due to alcohol, and about 7% of alcohol drinkers have moderate levels of dependency symptoms. Alcohol abuse can damage brain cells, the liver, and other vital organs. It also increases the risk of cancer, heart disease, high blood pressure, and nervous disorders. Substance abuse of any kind can lead to violence or accidents.

Clearly, many Americans are not fit and pay for it with poor health. How do law enforcement officers measure up to the general population?

Officers' Fitness

There are no national databases that allow for a comprehensive assessment of fitness levels, but for some years the Cooper Institute for Aerobics Research in Dallas, Texas, has been measuring the physical performance of various populations. Their data on more than 30,000 subjects are generally accepted as representative of the U.S. population as a whole, and are often used as a point of reference when evaluating physical performance. Let's consider some studies that compare law enforcement performance against these data.

The first attempt to draw some inferences about officer fitness was the 1977 study conducted for the International Association of Chiefs of Police (IACP). For a sample of 203 officers, cardiorespiratory endurance levels and percent body fat approached only the 25th percentile of the general population (75% of the general population scored better). Upper body and abdominal strength were between the 20th and 35th percentiles. Flexibility scores were at the 45th percentile. These figures suggest that the officers studied were fatter and weaker and had less stamina and flexibility than the general population they were responsible to safeguard.

One of the populations that the Cooper Institute has studied is law enforcement officers. From 1983 to 1992, they found some improvement in baseline fitness. Officers' aerobic fitness approached the 35th percentile of the general population, with fat at the 30th percentile. Upper body strength and flexibility were approximately at the 50th percentile, with abdominal strength at the 40th.

The most recent study was the 1992 Penn State Aging Study that collected data for 5,000 to 10,000 officers in six large agencies. The results of this survey suggest that officers are below average in aerobic fitness and body fat but somewhat above average in strength and lower-back flexibility.

For all these studies, officers over 35 years old scored worse against their civilian peers than did younger officers. Special units such as SWAT teams had the highest fitness levels.

These data suggest two things. First, officers are generally in poorer physical condition than their civilian contemporaries. Second, they compare even less favorably the longer they are on the force. Why is this?

First, there is little day-to-day physical activity in their jobs. Unlike a lumberjack, for example, whose work keeps him fit, an officer must develop physical fitness off of the job. In addition, irregular hours and unpredictable meal schedules can contribute to poor nutrition. Finally, a number of aspects of the job contribute to stress: the potential danger, the need to switch from inaction to action quickly, the necessity of dealing with people who are upset or angry, or even inactivity itself. Many choose to deal with these stressors by overeating, smoking, or abusing alcohol. All of these factors taken together can create a vicious circle from which it becomes difficult to escape. These lifestyle choices affect not only performance but health as well.

Officers' Health

It is virtually impossible to discuss fitness without mentioning its health implications. Research findings have consistently shown a link between lifestyle and disease. What you eat, whether you smoke, how much you drink, how you deal with stress, and your physical fitness all have a direct bearing on health as well as job performance.

Mortality statistics suggest that law enforcement officers have increased risk of premature death and may have a special vulnerability for certain diseases. Most studies indicate that law enforcement officers die at earlier ages than expected for the general population for all causes of death, and in particular for diabetes, colon cancer, and cardiovascular disease. Studies also show that law enforcement officers have a higher suicide rate than the general population. This may be linked to the amount of stress associated with the work.

The Cooper studies examined medical histories of law enforcement officers for medical problems. These officers represented small, medium, and large local, state, and federal agencies. The resulting data, summarized in Table 1.1, showed what percentages of incumbents had major medical problems.

Survey data indicate that only 80% of officers reach scheduled retirement. Fourteen percent take early retirement due to medical problems, and 6% die while employed as law enforcement officers. Even among the retired officers, a large percentage are in some sort of disability status. For example, the California Peace Officers Association reports that 73% of all officers who retire in that state do so due to a disability (*Law & Order*, May 1994, p. 70).

Professional groups such as the International Association for Chiefs of Police (IACP) and the Commission on Accreditation for Law Enforcement Agencies (CALEA), as well as many state peace officer standards and training councils, have recognized that fitness and health problems do exist, and have proposed policies in an attempt to alleviate their effects.

Benefits of a Fitness Program

So far you've seen some of the negative impacts that lack of fitness can cause. Here are some of the personal benefits of an effective fitness program.

Improved Job Performance

Studies have found that more physically fit officers generally receive higher job performance ratings. There are additional job performance benefits.

Improved Performance of Essential Physical Tasks

For the unfit, this improvement may equate to satisfactory performance in areas which were previously below par. For the already fit, it may mean improving already satisfactory performance to an even higher level.

Reduced Likelihood of Excessive Force

More fit, confident officers are less likely to be involved in use-of-force situations for several reasons. A suspect may think twice about physically challenging a more fit officer. A

Table 1.1 Percentage of Incumbents With Major Medical Problems	
Medical problem	**Percentage**
Obesity/overweight	20-50%
High cholesterol	20-35%
Orthopedic and back injuries	15-25%
Psychological problems	8-25%
Heart disease	5-10%
Gastrointestinal	5-10%
Hypertension	4-15%
Diabetes	1-2%

Note. Data from Collingwood (1988, 1993), IACP (1977), and McHenry et al. (1972).

more fit officer may be able to meet a physical challenge without resorting to the next level of force, e.g., going from grappling to using a baton. Finally, the more fit officer is likely to overcome a suspect on foot and avoid having to use more force than necessary to stop someone fleeing the scene.

Health Benefits

In addition to improved performance, you are likely to see the following health benefits.

Prevention of Health Problems

Better fitness not only restores health but also prevents health problems from developing. For example, regular vigorous physical activity helps prevent coronary heart disease and assists in weight control. Exercise that builds muscular strength and endurance and develops flexibility may protect against injury and disability. Physical activity also can bring about changes that help prevent and control hypertension (high blood pressure), heart disease, and diabetes.

Longer Life

Better fitness can also contribute to longevity. In a study of 16,936 Harvard alumni over a 16-year period, those who expended at least 2,000 calories per week in physical activity had a 28% lower risk of death from any cause.

Better Daily Living

Better fitness can improve people's daily lives. Participants in fitness programs have less fatigue and greater productivity. Regular exercise also has been shown to help reduce anxiety and tension and reduce cardiovascular reactions to stress. And the latest research is demonstrating that fitness can help prevent depression and anxiety and increase self-esteem.

Less Risk of Disability

You've worked hard in your profession, and certainly look forward to a well-deserved retirement. The numbers show that many of your colleagues are unable to enjoy their retirement years fully because of health problems which are directly related to lifestyle choices. Making changes in your lifestyle now can help ensure that you enjoy what you have worked so hard for.

Organizational Benefits

The following benefits are common among workers involved in a fitness program.

Fewer Sick Days

Fit and active employees have lower absenteeism rates. Companies report 20%-35% reductions in absenteeism after the installation of a worksite program. Studies performed with law enforcement officers indicate that the more fit and active officers, especially over age 35, have lower absenteeism rates. Some report 29% to 42% less absenteeism for fit and active officers compared to sedentary officers. One agency reported an 87% drop in sick time due to job-related injuries.

Improved Productivity

Fitness and productivity tend to be positively related. Data from occupations such as salespeople, textile workers, and office workers indicate that active workers have higher productivity. Studies performed with law enforcement officers, wherein supervisors' ratings of performance were analyzed, indicate that the more fit and active officers obtain higher ratings.

Reduced Health Care Costs

Preliminary data suggest that the introduction of a worksite fitness program reduces worker health care costs. Several studies found that medical expenses dropped for participating and active employees. Lower agency health care costs mean more money for your agency to spend in other areas, such as training programs, salaries, and benefits.

After reading this chapter, some of you might recognize that you need to do something about your fitness. Others of you may feel that your fitness level is adequate. Still others may not have a clue as to your status. Chapter 2 will help give you an idea of where you stand. You can assess your status in several fitness areas, and the results will give you a starting point for your new lifestyle.

CHAPTER 2

How Fit Are You?

As noted in chapter 1, you may already either recognize that you need a fitness program or feel comfortable that your fitness level is satisfactory, or you may just be unsure where you stand. In any case, the assessment instruments used in this chapter will give you a more precise determination of your fitness status.

Some of you will be reading this book to develop your own fitness program, and others will be using it under the guidance of a Fitness Coordinator or Instructor. This chapter may not be applicable for the latter group right now. It might be a good idea, however, to familiarize yourself with its content in case someday you need to develop a program, either for yourself or for someone else. It may also help you to understand your agency's assessment process a little better. For those reasons, this chapter includes examples of officers whose agencies do have fitness testing.

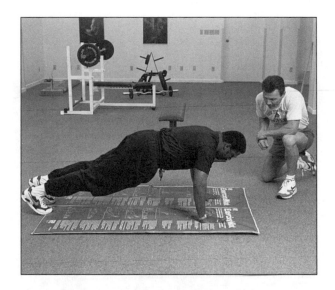

Screening Before Testing

Strenuous or even moderate exercise can be risky for some people with certain health problems. That's why it's essential that you undergo screening for such health problems before you begin fitness testing and an exercise program. Screening can identify whether you are likely to have a problem and thus need to see a doctor before you begin.

The Preparticipation Checklist in Figure 2.1 is a self-administered screening tool named PAR-Q. It will identify those who should consult with a doctor before beginning an exercise program. Answer each question "yes" or "no."

If there are any "yes" answers, you should see a doctor before attempting the physical fitness assessment shown later in this chapter or beginning an exercise program.

When you finish this chapter, you will be able to:

✪ Understand the precautions necessary before taking a fitness test or beginning a fitness program.

✪ Recognize different types of assessments (fitness tests).

✪ Determine your current fitness status by using the assessment tools presented in this chapter.

The PAR-Q is a good screening tool and easy to administer. Yet there are other indicators of your relative risk for exercise. The following information is included for those whose concerns about their risk of exercise persist after reviewing the PAR-Q.

While no set of guidelines can cover every possible scenario, the American College of Sports Medicine (ACSM) has studied this matter in detail. They have identified three classifications for individuals considering either exercise testing or increasing their level of physical activity.

■ Apparently healthy—those who have no symptoms or complaints, appear to be healthy, and have no more than one of the major coronary risk factors shown in Table 2.1.

■ Individuals at higher risk—those who have two or more major coronary risk factors (Table 2.1), and/or symptoms sugges-

Table 2.1
Major Coronary Risk Factors
1. Diagnosed hypertension or systolic blood pressure ≥ 160 or diastolic blood pressure ≥ 90 mmHg on at least two separate occasions, or on antihypertension medication.
2. Serum cholesterol ≥ 240 mg/dl
3. Cigarette smoking
4. Diabetes mellitus
5. Family history of coronary or other atherosclerotic disease in parents or siblings prior to age 55

Note. From Guidelines for Exercise Testing and Prescription (4th ed.) (p. 6) by the American College of Sports Medicine, 1991, Philadelphia: Lea & Febiger. Copyright 1991 by Williams & Wilkins. Reprinted by permission.

Table 2.2
Major Symptoms or Signs Suggestive of Cardiopulmonary or Metabolic Disease
1. Pain or discomfort in the chest or surrounding areas.
2. Unaccustomed shortness of breath or shortness of breath with mild exertion
3. Dizziness or faintness
4. Difficulty in breathing
5. Ankle swelling
6. Rapid heart rate
7. Swelling in the lower legs
8. Known heart murmur

Note. From Guidelines for Exercise Testing and Prescription (4th ed.) (p. 6) by the American College of Sports Medicine, 1991, Philadelphia: Lea & Febiger. Copyright 1991 by Williams & Wilkins. Reprinted by permission.

	Yes	No
1. Has a doctor ever said that you have heart trouble?	____	____
2. Do you suffer frequently from chest pains?	____	____
3. Do you often feel faint or have spells of severe dizziness?	____	____
4. Has a doctor ever said your blood pressure was too high?	____	____
5. Has a doctor ever told you that you have a bone or joint problem, such as arthritis, that has been or could be aggravated by exercise?	____	____
6. Are you over age 65 and not accustomed to any exercise?	____	____
7. Are you taking any prescription medications, such as those for heart problems or high blood pressure?	____	____
8. Is there a reason not mentioned here that you should not follow an exercise program?	____	____

Figure 2.1 *Preparticipation checklist.*
Note. From "PAR-Q Validation Report (modified version) by the British Columbia Department of Health" by D.M. Chisholm, M.L. Collins, L.L. Kulak, W. Davenport, and N. Gruber. Reprinted from the British Columbia Medical Journal 1975; 17:11.

tive of possible cardiopulmonary (heart and lung) or metabolic disease (Table 2.2). Metabolic disease includes diabetes mellitus, thyroid disorders, renal disease, and liver disease.

■ Individuals with disease—those with known cardiac, pulmonary, or metabolic disease.

The ACSM says that an examination such as a treadmill test is desirable for all persons over 45 years old before starting a vigorous exercise program and for higher-risk individuals of any age. For those without symptoms, it may not be necessary if moderate exercise is undertaken gradually with appropriate guidance and no competitive participation.

The ACSM recommends a thorough medical evaluation for all individuals with known cardiovascular, pulmonary, or metabolic disease. It is important to assess the safety of vigorous exercise and provide a baseline so that progress can be monitored.

Agency Fitness Testing

Depending on your agency's fitness program, you may be tested periodically for fitness. If so, you already have an idea of your fitness status. Depending on your score on each event, chapter 13 will give you guidance on setting goals appropriate to your level of fitness.

Most law enforcement agencies administer either a physical fitness test or a job task simulation test. Fitness tests measure the components of physical fitness discussed in chapter 1. A typical fitness test is the National Law Enforcement Fitness Test, also known as the Cooper Test. It consists of a 12-minute or 1.5-mile run (cardiovascular endurance), bench press and leg press (muscular strength), sit-ups and push-ups (muscular endurance), sit-and-reach (flexibility), 300-meter run (anaerobic power), and skinfold measurements (body fat). These components of fitness underlie all physical tasks performed by law enforcement officers.

Job task simulation tests, sometimes called ability or agility tests, consist of a series of physical tasks that law enforcement officers would typically perform. You might think of it as an obstacle course. For example, a test may be run over a 300-meter course which includes climbing a fence, jumping over a culvert, and dragging a weighted dummy. One drawback of job task simulation tests is that a typical battery accounts for only 20%-25% of the physical tasks performed by law enforcement officers.

Regardless of which type of test your agency has, the more important factor is a fitness program. The test can give you a starting point for your program and evaluate the effectiveness of the program, but the program itself is what makes you perform your job better.

Assessing Your Fitness Level

If you don't have a test in your agency, the following fitness assessment is relatively simple to administer and score. It is simpler than the seven-item test, which requires a trained supervisor to administer, but will nevertheless give you enough information about your fitness level to start a program. To complete the assessment, you will need a stopwatch, a box, a yardstick, and a track or other area to walk or run a known distance. Your local high school probably has a quarter-mile track, and that would be a good place to do the test. Record your results on the physical fitness assessment sheet shown in Figure 2.2. (You might want to make copies of this form to record your progress on retests.)

Screening Tests

Screening Tests are baseline measurements that are used to monitor your progress throughout your training program.

Name: _____		
Screening tests		
1. Height	_____	in.
2. Weight	_____	lbs
3. Resting heart rate	_____	beats/min
4. Resting blood pressure	_____	mm/Hg
5. Cholesterol (if available)	_____	mg/dl
Fitness tests		
Test	Score	Fitness category
1. 1.5-mile run	_____	_____
2. Sit-up	_____	_____
3. Push-up	_____	_____
4. Sit-and-reach	_____	_____
5. 1-mile walk ($\dot{V}O_2$max)	_____	_____

Figure 2.2 *Physical fitness assessment sheet.*

1. *Height.* Take this measurement in your stocking feet. Your fitness program won't change this measurement, but you'll use your height later to determine your Body Mass Index, which is an estimate of how much body fat you have.

2. *Weight.* Weigh yourself wearing as little clothing as you are comfortable with, and try to dress the same for subsequent weighings.

3. *Resting heart rate.* Sit quietly for at least 5 minutes before taking this measurement. You will need a stopwatch or a watch with a sweep second hand. Locate your pulse in one of two places (see Figure 2.3): your carotid pulse, to the side of your throat; or, your radial pulse, on the thumb side off the center line of your wrist. Don't use your thumb to take your pulse because it has a pulse if its own, which will confuse your count. Start your count on a beat with "zero," and continue for 60 seconds.

4. *Resting blood pressure.* If you can get someone to take your resting blood pressure, it is useful information. Many drugstores have machines which measure blood pressure. As a minimum, you'll want to compare it with the ACSM guideline for exercise participation of 160/90.

5. *Cholesterol screening.* Your agency may offer cholesterol screening. If not, local outpatient clinics and public health agencies often provide this service inexpensively.

You will learn how to perform the *fitness tests* in the pages to follow. Enter the raw score for each event in the space indicated in Figure 2.2. Refer to Table 2.3 (pp. 19-20) for the fitness categories, and record them in the space provided.

Before starting the test battery, you will have completed your screening and obtained clearance from your doctor if necessary. You should avoid eating or smoking for at least 1 hour before beginning the test battery. If possible, get someone to help you with the test. You can administer it to yourself, but it will be easier if you have help.

Always warm up before physical activity. As a minimum, jog easily until you break a sweat. Then do about 5 minutes of stretching exercises, concentrating on the body parts to be exercised. See chapter 6 for more information about warm-up.

Try to do the entire test battery in 1 day. If that's not possible, be sure to eventually complete each event so you have a starting point for your program. Figure 2.4 gives a recommended sequence of events and time schedule for the test battery.

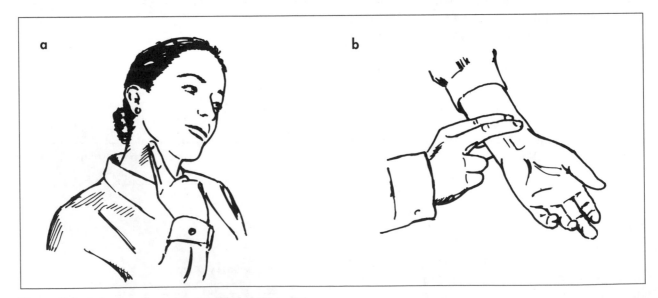

Figure 2.3 *Pulse locations: (a) carotid and (b) radial.*

One-Minute Sit-Up Test

Purpose

This test measures the endurance of the abdominal muscles. This is important for performing tasks that involve the use of force, and it helps maintain good posture and minimize lower-back problems. The score is in the number of sit-ups completed in 1 minute. This test should be performed on grass, a mat, or a carpeted surface. As a training vehicle, curl-ups are better but are difficult to test.

Equipment

- A mat, if desired
- A stopwatch
- A helper

Procedures

1. Lie on your back, knees bent, heels flat on the mat or ground. Hands should be held behind the head, with elbows out to the sides. Your partner should hold your feet down. If a helper is not available, put your feet under a couch or similar item to hold them down.

2. Perform as many correct sit-ups as possible in 1 minute. In the up position, you must touch your elbows to your knees and then return to a full lying position before starting the next sit-up. You may rest in either the starting or up position. See Figure 2.5 for the correct positions.

1.	Warm up 5-10 minutes
2.	1-minute sit-up test
3.	Rest 5 minutes
4.	Maximum push-up test
5.	Rest 5 minutes
6.	Sit-and-reach test
7.	Rest 10 minutes
8.	1-mile walk or 1.5-mile run
9.	Cool down 5 minutes

Figure 2.4 *Recommended sequence and time schedule.*

3. The score is the number of correct sit-ups. Record the score on the physical fitness assessment sheet (Figure 2.2, p. 13).

Maximum Push-Up Test

Purpose

This test measures the muscular endurance of certain upper body muscles. It is important for use-of-force situations which involve a pushing motion.

Equipment

- A stopwatch
- A helper, if available

Procedures

1. Get down on the floor into the front leaning rest position. Put your palms on the ground, approximately shoulder-width apart, back straight, feet approximately 8" apart.

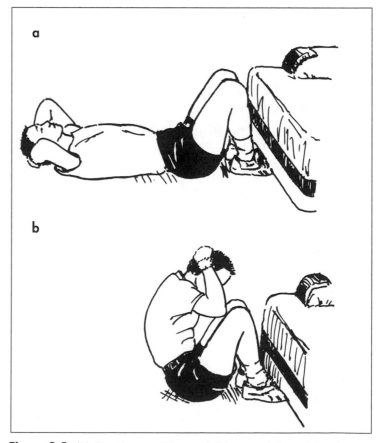

Figure 2.5 *(a) Starting position and (b) up position of the sit-up.*

2. If you have a helper, that person should crouch in front of you and ensure that your upper arms are parallel to the ground each time you lower yourself before returning to the starting position.

3. Lower your body by bending your elbows until your upper arms are parallel to the ground, then push up again. Keep your back straight, and in each extension up, lock the elbows out. See Figure 2.6 for pictures of the correct positions.

4. Rest in the up position.

5. Record the score on the physical fitness assessment sheet (Figure 2.2, p. 13). The score is the number of correct push-ups completed.

Sit-and-Reach Test

Purpose

This test measures the flexibility of the lower back and upper leg area, which is important for performing tasks involving range of motion and in minimizing lower-back problems. The score is recorded in inches to the nearest half.

Equipment

■   A 12"-high box

■   A yardstick attached to the top of the box, with the 15" mark at the edge of the box, and the 36" mark pointing away from you

■   A helper (mandatory)

Procedures

1. Warm up slowly by practicing the test.

2. Sit on the ground or mat with your shoes off and your legs extended at right angles to the box. Keep the legs straight. The heels touch the near edge of the box and are 8" apart. The yardstick is centered over the space between your legs.

3. Slowly reach forward with both hands (one on top of the other) as far as possible and hold the position momentarily. Have your helper note the distance reached on the yardstick by the fingertips to the nearest half inch. See Figure 2.7 for correct execution of the sit-and-reach.

4. The best of three trials is your score. Record your score on the physical fitness assessment sheet.

One-Mile Walk

If you have been inactive for a period of time, or if it was recommended by your doctor, assess your cardiovascular fitness with the 1-mile-walk test outlined here.

Purpose

This test is recommended only for officers who, because of an acute injury, inactivity, or very poor fitness, cannot take the 1.5-mile run. This test enables individuals who can not or should not run to obtain an estimate of

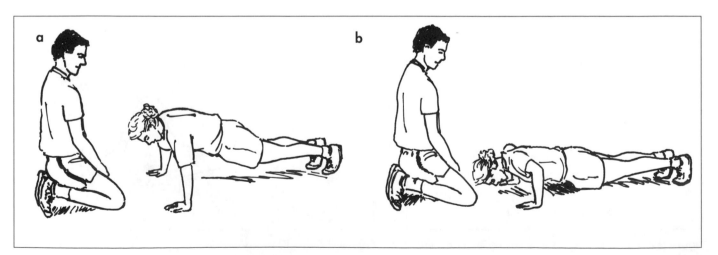

Figure 2.6 *(a) Starting position and (b) down position of the push-up.*

their cardiovascular fitness. (Cardiovascular fitness is estimated by the maximum amount of oxygen the body can use in a given period of time. This is referred to as "$\dot{V}O_2$max.")

Equipment

- Stopwatch
- 440-yard track or marked level course

Procedures

Before testing, determine an accurately measured course of exactly 1 mile. A one-quarter-mile running track is ideal.

1. Walk 1 mile as fast as possible. Running or jogging is not permitted.

2. When you finish the mile, note your time and immediately find either your radial or carotid pulse. Take the pulse for 6 seconds, and multiply the count by 10. (It is critical that you record your pulse as soon as you cross the finish line in order to get an accurate exercise heart rate.)

3. Cool down by walking slowly for 5 minutes.

4. Using your weight, age, sex, 1-mile-walk time, and 1-mile-walk heart rate, you can obtain a good estimate of your $\dot{V}O_2$max by using the following formula:

   $\dot{V}O_2$max = 132.853 - (0.0769 x WT) - (0.3877 x AGE) + (6.315 x SEX) - (3.2649 x T) - (0.1565 x HR),

   where WT = weight in pounds, AGE = age in years, SEX = 0 (for female) or 1 (for male), T = walk time in minutes to the nearest tenth, and HR = heart rate at the end of the walk.

   Example: A 190-pound, 40-year-old male walks the mile in 12:45, and gets a 6-second pulse count of 14 at the end of the walk (14 x 10 = 140 beats/min).

   $\dot{V}O_2$max= 132.853 - (0.0769 x 190) - (0.3877 x 40) + (6.315 x 1) - (3.2649 x 12.7) - (0.1565 x 140) = 132.853 – 14.611 – 15.508 + 6.315 - 41.464 - 21.91 = 51.394

5. Compare the estimate with norms for $\dot{V}O_2$max in Table 2.3 to determine fitness category.

6. Record the score on the physical fitness assessment sheet (Figure 2.2, p. 13).

1.5-Mile Run

Purpose

This run is a measure of cardiovascular endurance or aerobic power.

Equipment

- 440-yard track or marked level course
- Stopwatch
- A helper, if available

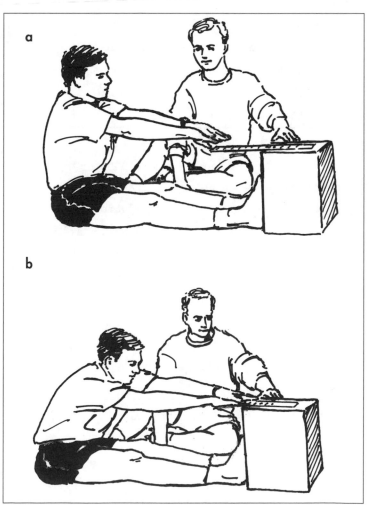

Figure 2.7 *(a) Starting position and (b) down position of the sit-and-reach.*

Procedures

Before testing, determine an accurately measured course of exactly 1 mile. A one-quarter-mile running track is ideal.

1. Warm up and stretch before the run.

2. If you have a helper, have the helper give the command "go" and begin timing. If not, start the watch yourself as you begin running.

3. Run the distance as fast as possible. Note your time at the end of the run.

4. Cool down by walking for an additional 5 minutes or so. Cooling down helps speed up the return of blood to the heart, reducing the chance of fainting. (See more on warm-up and cool-down in chapter 6.)

5. The score is the time it takes to run the course. Record the score on the physical fitness assessment sheet (Figure 2.2, p. 13).

Once you have finished the test and have recorded the results, compare them with the norms in Table 2.3. These tables are arranged by age and gender. Find your score in the appropriate table, determine your fitness category for each event, and write it in the appropriate space on the physical fitness assessment sheet.

Sample Test Results

Consider the performance results of Officer Hernandez, whose agency has mandatory testing but voluntary participation. When Tony went to his agency's Fitness Coordinator for help, the Coordinator pulled out the results of Tony's most recent assessment. Not surprisingly, the test scores were not very good. But they gave the coordinator a starting point for prescribing a fitness program for Tony. Look at Tony's scores in Figure 2.8.

Because Tony's agency administers the seven-item test, his results are more extensive than someone who just uses the four events for the self-assessment.

You'll see how the sample officers used the assessment results to establish goals and develop a program in subsequent chapters. Now that you have a feel for your current level of fitness, you will learn more about each component of physical fitness and how to develop a program to help you improve your performance in your weak areas.

Name: Tony Hernandez		
Screening tests		
1. Height		70 in.
2. Weight		230 lbs
3. Resting heart rate		84 beats/min
4. Resting blood pressure		145/95 mmHg
5. Step test		150 b/m
Fitness tests		
1. Percent fat		33% fat
2. Sit-up		22 repetitions
3. 1RM bench press	pounds	200 lbs
	ratio	.87 ratio
4. Push-up		10 repetitions
5. 300-meter run		Did not finish
6. Sit-and-reach		13 in.
7. 1RM leg press	pounds	270 lbs
	ratio	1.17 ratio
8. Run/walk	1.5-mile run	17:54 minutes/seconds
	12-minute run	___ X ___ miles/1/10ths

Figure 2.8 *Physical fitness assessment for Officer Hernandez.*

	Table 2.3				
	Assessment Norms: Females				

AGES 20-29

	1.5-mile run	**$\dot{V}O_2$max**	**Push-ups**	**Sit-ups**	**Sit-and-reach**
Superior (95-100%)	≤10:47	≥46.7	≥42	≥51	≥24
Excellent (80-94%)	10:48-12:20	41.0-46.6	28-41	45-50	23
Good (60-79%)	12:21-14:24	36.7-40.9	21-27	38-44	20-22
Fair (40-59%)	14:25-15:26	33.7-36.6	15-20	32-37	19
Poor (20-39%)	15:27-16:33	30.6-33.6	10-14	27-31	17-18
Very poor (0-19%)	≥16:34	≤30.5	≤9	≤26	≤16

AGES 30-39

	1.5-mile run	**$\dot{V}O_2$max**	**Push-ups**	**Sit-ups**	**Sit-and-reach**
Superior (95-100%)	≤11:49	≥43.8	≥40	≥42	≥24
Excellent (80-94%)	11:50-13:06	38.6-43.7	23-39	37-41	23
Good (60-79%)	13:07-15:08	34.6-38.5	15-22	29-36	20-22
Fair (40-59%)	15:09-15:57	32.3-34.5	11-14	25-28	18-19
Poor (20-39%)	15:58-17:14	28.7-32.2	8-10	20-24	16-17
Very poor (0-19%)	≥17:15	≤28.6	≤7	≤19	≤15

AGES 40-49

	1.5-mile run	**$\dot{V}O_2$max**	**Push-ups**	**Sit-ups**	**Sit-and-reach**
Superior (95-100%)	≤14:20	≥41.0	≥20	≥37	≥22
Excellent (80-94%)	14:21-15:29	36.3-40.9	16-19	32-36	21
Good (60-79%)	15:30-16:58	32.3-36.2	12-15	24-31	19-20
Fair (40-59%)	16:59-17:54	29.4-32.2	9-11	20-23	17-18
Poor (20-39%)	17:55-18:49	26.5-29.3	6-8	14-19	15-16
Very poor (0-19%)	≥18:50	≤26.4	≤5	≤13	≤14

AGES 50-59

	1.5-mile run	**$\dot{V}O_2$max**	**Push-ups**	**Sit-ups**	**Sit-and-reach**
Superior (95-100%)	≤14:20	≥36.8	≥15	≥30	≥23
Excellent (80-94%)	14:21-15:29	32.3-36.7	11-14	26-29	21-22
Good (60-79%)	15:30-16:58	29.4-32.2	7-10	20-25	18-20
Fair (40-59%)	16:59-17:54	26.8-29.3	3-6	14-19	16-17
Poor (20-39%)	17:55-18:49	24.3-26.7	1-2	10-13	14-15
Very poor (0-19%)	≥18:50	≤24.2	Ø	≤9	≤13

AGES ≥60

	1.5-mile run	**$\dot{V}O_2$max**	**Push-ups**	**Sit-ups**	**Sit-and-reach**
Superior (95-100%)	≤14:06	≥37.4	≥10	≥28	≥23
Excellent (80-94%)	14:07-15:57	31.2-37.3	7-9	19-27	19-22
Good (60-79%)	15:58-17:46	27.2-31.1	4-6	11-18	17-18
Fair (40-59%)	17:47-18:44	24.5-27.1	2-3	5-10	15-16
Poor (20-39%)	18:45-19:21	22.7-24.4	1	3-4	13-14
Very poor (0-19%)	≥19:22	≤22.6	Ø	≤2	≤12

Note. Data from the Cooper Institute for Aerobics Research, Dallas, TX.

Table 2.3
Assessment Norms: Males

AGES 20-29

	1.5-mile run	$\dot{V}O_2$max	Push-ups	Sit-ups	Sit-and-reach
Superior (95-100%)	≤8:13	≥54	≥62	≥55	≥23
Excellent (80-94%)	8:14-9:45	48.2-53.9	51-61	49-54	21-22
Good (60-79%)	9:46-11:41	44.2-48.1	37-50	42-48	18-20
Fair (40-59%)	11:42-12:51	41.0-44.1	29-36	38-41	16-17
Poor (20-39%)	12:52-14:13	37.1-40.9	22-28	33-37	14-15
Very poor (0-19%)	≥14:14	≤37.0	≤21	≤32	≤13

AGES 30-39

	1.5-mile run	$\dot{V}O_2$max	Push-ups	Sit-ups	Sit-and-reach
Superior (95-100%)	≤8:44	≥52.5	≥52	≥51	≥22
Excellent (80-94%)	8:45-10:16	46.8-52.4	41-51	45-50	20-21
Good (60-79%)	10:17-12:20	42.4-46.7	30-40	39-44	17-19
Fair (40-59%)	12:21-13:36	38.9-42.3	24-29	35-38	15-16
Poor (20-39%)	13:37-14:52	35.3-38.8	17-23	30-34	13-14
Very poor (0-19%)	≥14:53	≤35.2	≤16	≤29	≤12

AGES 40-49

	1.5-mile run	$\dot{V}O_2$max	Push-ups	Sit-ups	Sit-and-reach
Superior (95-100%)	≤9:30	≥50.3	≥51	≥47	≥21
Excellent (80-94%)	9:31-11:18	44.1-50.2	28-50	40-46	19-20
Good (60-79%)	11:19-13:14	39.9-44.0	19-27	34-39	16-18
Fair (40-59%)	13:15-14:29	36.7-39.8	13-18	29-33	14-15
Poor (20-39%)	14:30-15:41	33.0-36.6	9-12	24-28	12-13
Very poor (0-19%)	≥15:42	≤32.9	≤8	≤23	≤11

AGES 50-59

	1.5-mile run	$\dot{V}O_2$max	Push-ups	Sit-ups	Sit-and-reach
Superior (95-100%)	≤10:40	≥47.1	≥40	≥43	≥21
Excellent (80-94%)	10:41-12:20	41.0-47.0	34-39	36-42	18-20
Good (60-79%)	12:21-14:24	36.7-39.9	24-33	28-35	15-17
Fair (40-59%)	14:25-15:26	33.8-36.6	18-23	24-27	13-14
Poor (20-39%)	15:27-16:43	30.1-33.7	11-17	19-23	10-12
Very poor (0-19%)	≥16:44	≤30.0	≤10	≤18	≤9

AGES ≥60

	1.5-mile run	$\dot{V}O_2$max	Push-ups	Sit-ups	Sit-and-reach
Superior (95-100%)	≤11:20	≥45.2	≥28	≥39	≥20
Excellent (80-94%)	11:21-13:22	38.0-45.1	24-27	31-38	18-19
Good (60-79%)	13:23-15:29	33.6-37.9	18-23	22-30	14-17
Fair (40-59%)	15:30-16:43	30.1-33.5	10-17	19-21	12-13
Poor (20-39%)	16:44-18:00	26.5-30.0	6-9	15-18	10-11
Very poor (0-19%)	≥18:01	≤26.4	≤5	≤14	≤9

Note. Data from the Cooper Institute for Aerobics Research, Dallas, TX.

PART II

Physical Fitness

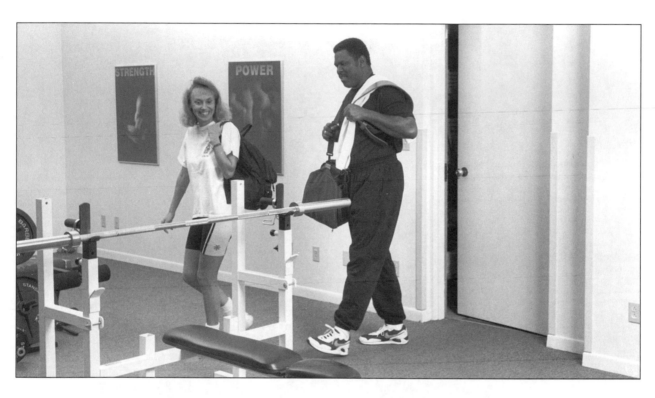

I n Part I you learned what the components of physical fitness are and assessed your own level of fitness. Now, you will learn more about the importance of the physical fitness components and how to train in each of the areas. When you finish this part of the book, you will have the knowledge needed to design an exercise program that will improve your cardiovascular endurance, anaerobic power, muscular strength and endurance, and flexibility. These activities, along with what you will learn later about diet and nutrition, will enable you to change your body composition, lowering the amount of fat and adding lean muscle mass. These improve-

ments will take time and require you to make changes in your behaviors, but will enhance your performance and health.

In chapter 3, we'll discuss the principles of exercise. The information about the principles of exercise applies equally well to the beginner and to more experienced fitness followers. In chapters 4 through 7, we'll discuss each of the components of physical fitness, and tell you how to train for each and what activities you use. You will learn the acronym "FITT," which will help you remember how to apply the principles of exercise to each component of physical fitness.

CHAPTER 3

Principles of Exercise

A s with other sciences, the science of exercise has principles which have been developed through observation and research and substantiated through practice.

The principles of exercise tell you how to exercise correctly and safely. You may see different combinations or lists in other fitness books, but the principles you'll learn here are selected for their appropriateness to law enforcement officers, although they could apply to any group of exercisers.

There are 11 principles of exercise to consider when designing your fitness program:

- Individuality
- Adaptation
- Overload
- Progression
- Specificity
- Regularity
- Recovery
- Balance
- Variety
- Reversibility
- Moderation

Principle #1: Individuality

Each person will respond somewhat differently to the same training routine. These dif-

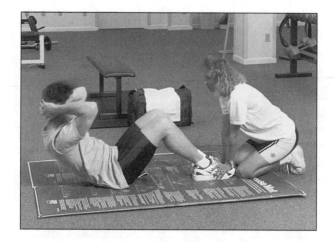

ferences are due to several factors, including heredity, eating and sleeping habits, the environment, illnesses and injuries, level of fitness, and motivation.

The principle of individuality means that some of you are more likely to become more fit in a cardiovascular way than you are to become really strong. Some are more likely to be good runners, others good swimmers, and yet others better bikers. And each of you has a different individual potential for how good you can be.

> **When you finish this chapter you will be able to:**
>
> ✪ Explain the principles of exercise.
>
> ✪ Understand the relationship of the principles of exercise to each other.
>
> ✪ Apply the principles of exercise to your fitness program.

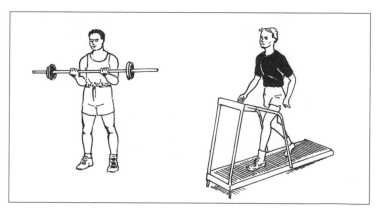

Principle #2: Adaptation

The body adjusts to the effects of training, but does it in small increments. Over time, these small increments cause major changes in your body. For example, the increases in muscle mass from strength training don't happen overnight. But one day you will discover that you need a new uniform because the old one doesn't fit the same way anymore. Only by comparing periodic measurements can you truly appreciate the day-to-day adaptations that are occurring. Understanding that fitness is a long-term investment is important to avoid frustration and disappointment.

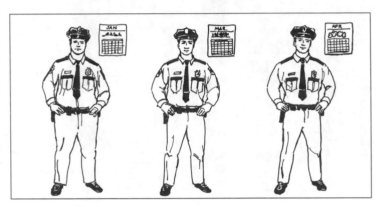

Principle #3: Overload

For a training program to have an effect, the demands placed on the body must be greater than those of your day-to-day activities. You'll never improve your cardiovascular endurance if your most strenuous exercise is walking from the patrol car to the station house (although a brisk walk might produce a

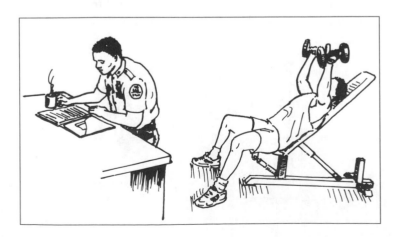

training effect). Nor will you increase your strength if you never overcome any more resistance than lifting a coffee cup. For each part of your program, as your fitness level improves you must increase the demands of your training to ensure overload.

Principle #4: Progression

There are two aspects of progression. One, as noted, is that as your level of fitness improves, you must increase the overload. The second is that these changes should be gradual. The story of the ancient Greek wrestler Milo illustrates both of these aspects. Milo trained in part by lifting a calf every day. As the calf grew into a cow, Milo's strength increased.

To improve your cardiovascular endurance, you must systematically train faster and/or longer. To improve your strength, you must increase the resistance your muscles must overcome. As your body adapts to the current overload, you must progressively increase that overload to continue to improve.

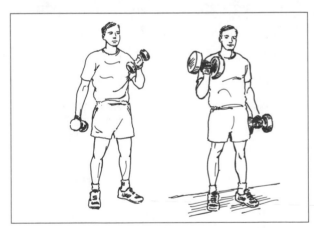

Principle #5: Specificity

Specificity in the fitness context means that you get good at what you practice. Running or other cardiovascular activities will not improve your muscular strength, and vice versa. It also means that you will show the greatest improvement in whatever activity you use for training. Running to improve your   cardiovascular   endurance   won't

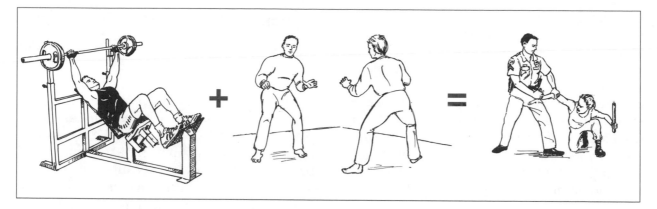

improve your swimming or cycling as much as it will your running ability.

Applying this principle to a law enforcement setting, let's consider strength and defensive tactics training. Getting stronger will help you perform better in a use-of-force situation. But the specific defensive tactics training will further improve that performance.

Principle #6: Regularity

The weekend-warrior approach to fitness training will probably produce more injuries than desirable results. To be effective, a fitness program must be followed regularly. Trying to get all the training you need in irregular bursts doesn't work. Rather, your training should be consistent throughout the week, the month, the year, and your life.

Fitness research indicates that it takes a minimum of three exercise sessions per week to achieve cardiovascular training. There are indications that as few as two strength sessions per week are necessary to see gains in

that area. As you will see later, you should do some flexibility training at least each time you do any exercise.

Compare fitness training to marksmanship training. If the only time you fire your weapon is during requalification, it is likely that your scores will go down. But if you have the opportunity to practice between qualifications, you are more likely to improve.

While it is important to train at least the minimum number of times for each of the fitness components each week, you don't want to overtrain.

Principle #7: Recovery

The body needs time to recover between hard exercise sessions. As a general rule, allow 48 hours for that recovery between hard exercise sessions. For example, if you lift weights for the upper body on Monday, you should wait until Wednesday before training those muscles again. However, working out the lower body on Tuesday will not violate this principle.

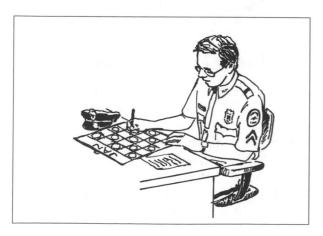

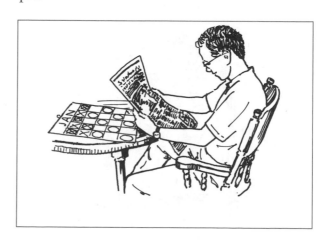

Along with recovering between exercise sessions, you need to get sufficient sleep and allow for recovery from peak physical events, such as your agency's fitness test or a race that you trained for. For most active people, getting 7 or 8 hours of sleep a night ensures sufficient rest for their lifestyle. When developing your long-range training plan, take into consideration that after an all-out effort, for which you have perhaps trained extra hard, you should go a little easier for a while.

Principle #8: Balance

To achieve total fitness, you must avoid concentrating on just one component. Sometimes people tend to concentrate on what they enjoy the most or do the best. Therefore, if you really enjoy running but don't enjoy strength training, you may tend to sacrifice the strength training and do more running. That's not bad, but you would be better off to do some training for all of the components of physical fitness.

Balance comes into play within each component as well. Some people who are into weightlifting, for example, may concentrate on certain parts of their bodies and ignore others.

The key is to have balance among the components of fitness and within each component. You may be the strongest officer in the agency, but if you have ignored your cardiovascular conditioning while concentrating on your strength, you may not be able to catch the suspect to subdue him.

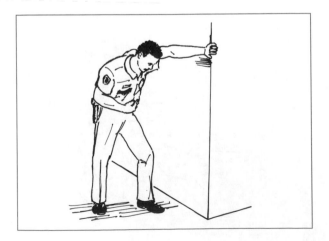

Principle #9: Variety

Variety ties in with balance, recovery, and specificity. Even the most die-hard fitness enthusiasts would get bored if they did the same exercises every day. Vary your routine to reduce the chance of boredom. For example, if you like to swim and have access to a pool, use both swimming and running to develop CVE and keep you excited about exercising. Find different places to train. Explore different weight training routines so that part of your program doesn't become stale.

As noted in the section on the principle of recovery, planning for rest is important. In fact, you can add variety to your program by periodically giving yourself an unexpected and unplanned day off.

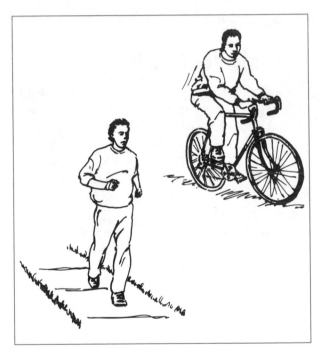

Principle #10: Reversibility

Most training adaptations are reversible. It takes longer to achieve a level of fitness than it does to lose it. Some setbacks in your training regimen are almost unavoidable. So the more "money in the bank" that you have stored up, the more able you will be to withstand those periods when you are unable to train. You must maintain your training.

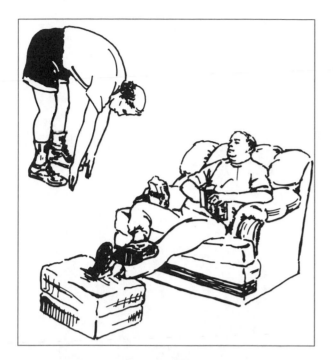

Principle #11: Moderation

Too much of anything can be bad. For best results, you must be dedicated to your program, but temper that dedication with common sense and good judgment. Don't train when you are injured. Also, more is not necessarily better. Too much distance, speed, weight, or time can all lead to deterioration rather than development. Moderation in all things, not just physical training, is a good rule for life.

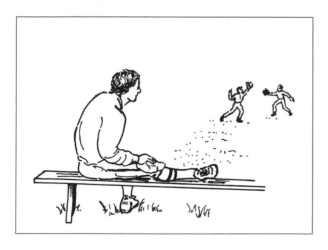

FITT

To design your fitness program, you must consider all the exercise principles. Most importantly, you need to know how often, how hard, and how long to exercise and what activities will produce a training effect. To help you remember this information, we will use the acronym FITT: Frequency, Intensity, Time, and Type of exercise.

In the next few chapters we will apply the principles of exercise to each of the components of physical fitness. You will learn FITT for each fitness component and will see more specifically how the principles relate to your training plan. It is not so important to memorize the list of principles. Instead, you merely need to understand the concepts they represent. That knowledge will ensure that your fitness program is safe and effective.

All of the information you need to develop a prescription for your fitness training can be summarized using the acronym FITT:

F — *Frequency.* How often to perform the type of exercise. Frequency incorporates the principles of regularity and recovery.

I — *Intensity.* How hard to exercise. Intensity incorporates the principles of overload and progression.

T — *Time.* How long the exercise session should be. Time also incorporates the principles of overload and progression.

T — *Type.* What types of activities train each component. Type incorporates the principles of specificity and variety.

CHAPTER 4

Cardiovascular Endurance

You probably use the word *energy* quite a bit, perhaps in phrases such as "I just don't have enough energy," or "I'm going to eat this candy bar to get an energy boost." Most people tend to attribute some nebulous quality to the term, but energy is a very real substance.

Certain foodstuffs stored in your bodies are released in the presence of oxygen to produce energy. This is called aerobic energy production. Quite simply, the process goes like this (see Figure 4.1). We breathe air into our lungs. There the oxygen passes into the bloodstream. The better trained our lungs are, the more oxygen is carried by the blood to working muscles. Some things we can control affect how well the blood carries the oxygen.

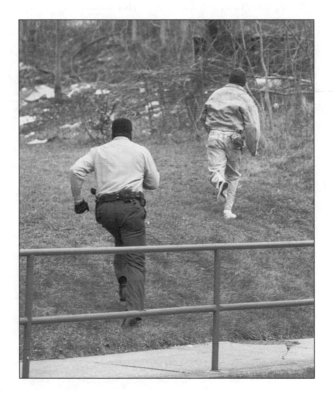

For example, alcohol blocks this ability, diminishing the amount of oxygen that reaches the working muscles.

Next, the oxygen passes from the bloodstream to the muscle where it combines with stored sugars to produce energy. The amount of sugar stored in the muscle and the efficiency of combining with oxygen are, once again, affected by training.

When the blood leaves the area of the muscle, it removes waste products of the energy production such as carbon dioxide. The training, which improves the different phases of this process, also improves cardiovascular endurance.

When you finish this chapter, you will be able to:

- ✪ Explain what cardiovascular endurance is and give examples of the types of activities that require it.

- ✪ Understand how the principles of exercise apply to cardiovascular endurance training.

- ✪ Develop an individual cardiovascular endurance training program.

- ✪ Know what activities you can participate in to improve your cardiovascular endurance.

- ✪ Begin a training program for this component of physical fitness.

What Is Cardiovascular Endurance?

As you learned in chapter 1, *cardiovascular endurance* is the ability to perform activity that requires the body to combine its energy sources with oxygen. It is essential for activities that require continuous effort for more than 2 minutes.

Cardiovascular endurance is important to both performance and health.

Law enforcement activities that require cardiovascular endurance include:

■ Foot pursuits

■ Use-of-force situations

Cardiovascular endurance is related to health because it:

■ Reduces risk of heart disease

■ Assists in controlling weight, particularly loss of excess body fat

■ Helps reduce stress

■ Reduces resting blood pressure

■ Raises levels of HDL—the good cholesterol

■ Helps regulate Type II diabetes mellitus

■ Helps prevent pulmonary disease

■ Delays onset of osteoporosis

■ Lowers risk of certain cancers, including colon and breast cancers

Designing Your Program

While each of the principles of fitness discussed in chapter 3 apply to cardiovascular endurance training, some of the applications are quite obvious and won't be discussed here. Instead, this discussion will concentrate on those that are most important in designing a cardiovascular endurance training program.

The program should address:

■ How often you should exercise

■ How hard to exercise

■ How long to exercise

■ The activity

To illustrate this, Officer Hernandez will serve as an example. As he answers each of these questions, he'll fill in this chart:

Frequency_____(number of workouts per week)

Intensity_____(how hard)

   Heart rate range _____
                                              (another measure of how hard)*

Time _____(duration of the workout)

Type _____(activity)

*Applies to cardiovascular endurance training program only.

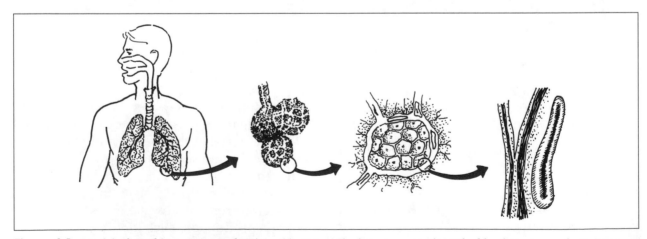

Figure 4.1 *Model of aerobic energy production. Air enters the lungs, passes into the bloodstream, and moves to the muscles, where it combines with stored sugars. Waste products such as carbon dioxide enter the bloodstream, return to the lungs, and are then exhaled.*

The principles of fitness most applicable to cardiovascular endurance training are:

- Overload
- Progression
- Specificity
- Regularity
- Recovery
- Variety

Overload

To understand this principle, consider the stress adaptation syndrome. According to Dr. Hans Selye, a recognized expert on the subject of stress, the body adjusts to the stressors it encounters in everyday life. Each time it makes these adaptations, it becomes better prepared to meet the next stressors—up to a point. If there is insufficient recovery time between each exposure to the stressors, they can overwhelm the body's ability to deal with them. That can cause unnecessary fatigue and injuries. But with sufficient recovery time, the body needs increasingly more difficult challenges in order to keep improving.

As a law enforcement officer, your day-to-day activities will not give you the cardiovascular endurance necessary for the occasional need to engage in a use-of-force situation, or to pursue a suspect. You need to "stress" the cardiovascular system with demands that are greater than your everyday activities in order to achieve a training effect.

Overload affects two components of FITT: intensity and time.

Intensity

Intensity refers to how hard the exercise should be. You will learn two ways to gauge the intensity of the workout. First is target heart rate (THR). This method uses the heart rate to estimate the intensity of your exercise. The heart rate increases during exercise. There is a correlation between the heart rate and the overload being placed on the cardiovascular system. To ensure that you are achieving the desired training effect, you must calculate your individual THR for the desired intensity. Because it is an estimate of the work you are doing, and because counting a rapid pulse can be difficult, we recommend that you establish a 20-beat target heart rate range for the THR.

There are several terms you will need to know in order to calculate your THR. Recall from chapter 2 that your resting heart rate (RHR) is how many times your heart beats in a minute while you are at rest. For the most accurate resting pulse, take it first thing in the morning before getting out of bed. That will also give you greater assurance that any variations you notice are due to changes in your body and not to changing conditions.

As your conditioning improves, you should see a gradual decline in the resting heart rate. If you see a sudden increase, it is probably caused by one of two things. You may be overtraining and need a rest, or you may be coming down with a cold or other ailment. You should also know that certain substances, for example caffeine and alcohol, will elevate your heart rate.

The maximum heart rate (MHR) is the greatest number of beats per minute that your heart is capable of. To predict MHR, subtract your age from 220. The estimated MHR for Officer Hernandez, who is 40 years old, for example, would be 220 - 40, or 180 beats per minute.

Assuming that Officer Hernandez could maximize his heart rate at 180, and given that his resting heart rate is 84, he has 96 beats "in reserve." That means he can perform activities that require up to 96 additional heartbeats per minute. This is his heart rate reserve (HRR).

The intensity of your workout will be at a certain percentage of your HRR. As noted earlier, one of the distinguishing features of CVE training is that it can be sustained over a period of time, so it cannot be an all-out effort. Depending on your fitness level and whether you are planning a hard or easy workout, we recommend that you train between 50% and 80% of your HRR.

Now that you know your RHR and MHR and understand that you will choose a percentage of your HRR at which to train, you are ready to calculate your training heart rate range. To do this, you will use what is known as the Karvonen formula. In Figure 4.2 we'll take a look at this calculation for Officer Hernandez, choosing a workout intensity of 50%.

When taking your pulse during exercise, only count it for 6 seconds, and multiply the count by 10. The heart rate drops very quickly when you stop exercising, so for a more accurate estimate, use the 6-second count. In our example, if Officer Hernandez' training heart rate was below 122, he would have to increase his pace to get the desired results. On the other hand, if it were over 142, he should slow down the pace.

Use the chart in Figure 4.3 to calculate your heart rate range for 50%, 60%, 70%, and 80% of your HRR. Remember that as your

---

1. To estimate maximal heart rate (MHR), subtract the individual's age from 220. (Officer Hernandez is 40.)

$$\begin{array}{rl} & 220 \\ - & 40 \quad \text{Age} \\ \hline & 180 \quad \text{MHR} \end{array}$$

2. Subtract the individual's resting heart rate (RHR) from the maximal heart rate to get the heart rate reserve (HRR). (Tony's RHR = 84.)

$$\begin{array}{rl} & 180 \\ - & 84 \quad \text{RHR} \\ \hline & 96 \quad \text{HRR} \end{array}$$

3. Multiply that number by the intensity [the percentage of the maximal heart rate (%MHR)] desired.

$$\begin{array}{rl} & 96 \\ \times & .50 \quad \text{MHR} \\ \hline & 48 \end{array}$$

4. Find the training heart rate (THR) by adding the resting heart rate to that number.

$$\begin{array}{rl} & 48 \\ + & 84 \quad \text{RHR} \\ \hline & 132 \quad \text{THR} \end{array}$$

5. Set the heart rate range by adding 10 beats below and 10 beats above the training heart rate. Target heart rate range =

$$\begin{array}{rl} & 132 \quad \text{THR} \\ \pm & 10 \\ \hline & 122\text{-}142 \end{array}$$

This tells him that to work at an intensity of 50% of his HRR, Officer Hernandez should keep his heart rate between 122 and 142 beats per minute.

Figure 4.2 *Example of calculating target heart rate range.*

---

1. Maximum heart rate (MHR) (220 - your age) _____

2. Resting heart rate (RHR) _____

3. Heart rate reserve (MHR - RHR = HRR) _____

4. HRR x .50 = _____ + RHR = _____ ± 10 = _____ to _____

5. HRR x .60 = _____ + RHR = _____ ± 10 = _____ to _____

6. HRR x .70 = _____ + RHR = _____ ± 10 = _____ to _____

7. HRR x .80 = _____ + RHR = _____ ± 10 = _____ to _____

Figure 4.3 *Calculating your training heart rate range.*

---

conditioning improves, your resting heart rate will drop, and so periodically you will have to recalculate these ranges.

The other method to estimate the intensity of your workout is the table of perceived exertion. A Swedish psychologist by the name of Borg established that peoples' perceptions of how hard they were working were surprisingly accurate. To use Table 4.1, simply answer the question, how does the exercise feel? The numbers in the right column, when multiplied by 10, will give you an estimate of your heart rate at the perceived level of exertion selected.

Time

The other element of overload is time or duration, that is, how long you must keep up the activity in order to achieve a training effect. As with intensity, duration varies according to your level of conditioning and your goals. It also varies with the type of workout. It is a variable that you can use to alter the results of the workout.

To achieve cardiovascular training, you need to train within your THR range for a minimum of 20 minutes. As your conditioning improves, you may increase this minimum. In general, as you increase the duration of the exercise, you will have to decrease the intensity in order to sustain the work for the desired length of time.

Officer Hernandez's fitness test results indicate that his level of conditioning is low. Therefore, he should start with no more than 20 minutes of exercise, if he can last that long.

Progression

The next principle to consider is progression, which also relates to the intensity and time components of FITT. Beginners should expect to see some improvements in about 3 weeks. Changes in more fit persons will come about more slowly. Plan to measure your cardiovascular fitness with the 1.5-mile run every 6 to 8 weeks, and adjust the intensity and duration accordingly. Remember, to continue to improve, you must increase the overload as your conditioning improves.

Table 4.1 Borg's Table of Perceived Exertion	
How does the exercise feel?	**Rating**
No exertion at all	6
Extremely light	7
	8
Very light	9
	10
Light	11
	12
Somewhat hard	13
	14
Hard (heavy)	15
	16
Very hard	17
	18
Extremely hard	19
Maximal exertion	20

Note. From *An Introduction to Borg's RPE-Scale* by G. Borg, 1985, Ithaca, NY: Mouvement Publications. Copyright 1985 by Gunnar Borg. Reprinted by permission.

Regarding Officer Hernandez's program, he should plan to progress in each of the elements you have seen so far in his training program. When three workouts a week become easy, he should increase to four. As his conditioning improves, he will find that he can increase the intensity to 60% of his HRR. These improvements will also enable him to increase the time he spends exercising to 25, then 30 minutes. These changes should be gradual, and continue until he has reached his goals.

You may also reach a level where further improvement is not necessary. If you then continue to work at the same overload, you will maintain your conditioning. Of course factors such as illness, injury, travel, and aging all can affect this conditioning.

Specificity

Another factor to consider when developing your training plan is whether or not you have a specific goal, as opposed to general conditioning. For example, if your agency adminis-

ters a fitness test, the goal of your cardiovascular training may be to meet the agency's standard. This is where the principle of specificity comes into play. If your agency's test includes a 1.5-mile run, your training plan should include running to improve cardiovascular fitness. While other types of cardiovascular training, such as swimming, will improve your endurance, they will not prepare you for the 1.5-mile run as well as running will.

Regularity

To improve cardiovascular fitness, you must participate in an appropriate activity, at the necessary intensity and duration, a minimum of three times a week. More fit persons will probably choose to exercise as often as five or six times per week. But, as you learned in chapter 3, adequate rest is important in order to avoid injury and to enhance the positive training effects.

Recovery

While regularity is important, more is not necessarily better. Without adequate rest, the body's systems and muscles will eventually break down. To apply this principle to cardiovascular training, follow these rules of thumb:

- For those just beginning a training program, alternate days of training with days of rest.

- For more advanced exercisers, avoid training hard on two consecutive days. "Hard" may refer to the intensity or the length of the workout. For example, if you choose running as your activity for cardiovascular fitness, and you train 5 days a week, you might schedule your training like this:

Sunday — long, hard

Monday — short, easy

Tuesday — short, hard (fast)

Wednesday — rest

Thursday — long, easy

Friday — short, hard

Saturday — rest

You should also consider scheduling days of rest after your agency's fitness test, after a road race, or after any all-out effort.

Officer Hernandez, with a low fitness level, should begin his program with 3 days of cardiovascular exercise a week.

Variety

The last principle to consider when planning your cardiovascular fitness training is variety. There are several different ways to apply this principle.

While the principle of specificity allows you to become good at what you practice, you still might want to vary the activities you use to improve or maintain your cardiovascular fitness. If your goal is general fitness, then combining running, biking, and swimming, for example, will reduce the boredom which may result from doing just one of the activities all of the time.

Even if you use only one cardiovascular activity, variety will spice up your training. If you run, choosing different routes, times of the day, and running partners will make the training more interesting.

Specificity and variety relate to the type of activities that can give you a training effect. Table 4.2 gives you choices of activities that will improve your cardiovascular fitness. The most important consideration in choosing an activity is whether you enjoy it or not.

Tony has decided to choose brisk walking and jogging for his cardiovascular endurance training. His completed cardiovascular training plan would look like this:

Frequency _____3 days per week, with a day of rest between each

Intensity _____50%

Heart rate range _____122–142 bpm

Time _____20 minutes

Type _____Brisk walking and jogging

Table 4.2 Cardiovascular Endurance Activities	
Brisk walking	Jogging
Running	Swimming
Cycling	Cross-country skiing
Rowing	Aerobic dance
Stair-stepping	

Environmental Guidelines

Environmental conditions can have a significant impact on exercise safety and performance. When a person trains, he or she adapts to training within a certain environment. If that environment changes, an adjustment period is required, normally 30 days, for the person to achieve full acclimatization. Generally, the more fit the individual, the quicker the acclimatization.

Heat and Humidity

Hot weather can cause medical problems and even death. Every part of the country has these conditions at some time of the year. Apply the hot weather training guidelines in Table 4.3 in your fitness program.

Cold

Cold can also cause medical problems and even death. It places a burden on the body for temperature regulation and circulation. Cold stress can affect either peripheral body parts, causing frostbite, or the central core, causing life-threatening hypothermia.

Apply the cold environment training guidelines shown in Table 4.4 in your training program.

Altitude

At higher elevations there is less oxygen in the air, so one must work harder to maintain a given level of activity. Altitude starts to have a major effect on the body between 5,000 and 7,000 feet. The body adapts to a higher altitude by developing more red blood cells so

Table 4.3 Hot Weather Training Guidelines
Water
Exercisers need continual replenishment of water to avoid heat stress problems. ■ Drink 8 to 10 glasses of water each day. ■ Drink as much as can be tolerated before, during, and after exercise. ■ Don't drink unnecessary special athletic drinks for electrolyte replacement; water gets to the muscles quicker. ■ Don't take salt tablets; they are unnecessary. ■ If your body weight drops by more than 3% in one day, drink two cups of water to replace each pound of water loss.
Clothing
Exercisers should wear clothing that allows maximal evaporation to occur. ■ Don't wear rubber or plastic suits. ■ Do wear loose clothing made of absorbent materials that absorb sweat away from the body. ■ Wear clothes with light colors to reflect heat. ■ Don't use oil-based sunscreen.
Training intensity
Exercisers should modify their training until they are partially acclimatized (after 7-10 days). ■ Don't expect to perform as well as normal. ■ Reduce intensity and duration. ■ Monitor heart rate frequently, as it may increase more rapidly than normal.
Monitoring conditions
Exercisers must monitor the weather conditions. ■ Try to go out during the coolest part of the day, often the early morning. ■ Evaluate the heat and humidity conditions to determine whether to exercise and, if so, how hard.

Table 4.4 Cold Weather Training Guidelines
Water and food
Exercisers need to keep their core temperature up. ■ Drink plenty of fluids. Dehydration is also a problem in cold weather. ■ Avoid drinking alcohol. ■ Eat plenty of carbohydrates. Because the cold raises the body's metabolism, fuel burns up more quickly.
Clothing
Exercisers need to dress warmly for protection, yet avoid sweating. ■ Avoid sweating by dressing in removable, loose-fitting layers. ■ Wear fabrics that draw moisture away from the body. ■ Wear an outer layer that is wind resistant. ■ Wear a hat and something to cover the neck. ■ Wear mittens rather than gloves, as the fingers stay warmer when in contact with each other.
Training intensity
Exercisers need to keep moving while outside. ■ Warm up well before exercising and cool down indoors. ■ Lower exercise intensity. ■ Keep moving!
Monitoring conditions
Exercisers must monitor the weather conditions. ■ Try to go out during the warmest part of the day, often early afternoon. ■ Evaluate the cold conditions to determine whether to exercise and, if so, how hard.

more of the limited oxygen can be distributed. Until that acclimatization occurs, any workload will be more demanding, so workout intensity should be decreased.

The major problem caused by altitude is altitude sickness, a condition that occurs when someone is physically active at an altitude he or she hasn't adapted to yet. Cold weather problems may also appear at higher altitudes.

Apply the altitude training guidelines shown in Table 4.5 in your fitness program.

Pollution

Pollution poses a similar problem to that of altitude: there is not enough oxygen in the air because of competing pollutants. This lack of oxygen makes exercise more difficult, and

Table 4.5
Altitude Training Guidelines

Water—Drink plenty of water before, during, and after exercise.

Clothing—Wear the same clothing as for cold weather.

Training intensity—Generally it needs to be lowered.

Monitoring conditions—Keep track of wind chill.

Table 4.6
Pollution Training Guidelines

Time of day—Don't schedule exercise between 7 and 10 a.m. and 4 and 7 p.m. during peak traffic periods.

Place—Attempt to exercise in a location with low pollution.

Reduce exposure—As the effects of pollution accumulate over time, limit outdoor exercise if possible.

breathing the pollutants is potentially harmful as well. Pollution also makes exercising uncomfortable because of eye, nose, and lung irritation.

Three main pollutants cause respiratory stress:

- Ozone, which reduces cardiovascular endurance

- Sulphur dioxide, which can narrow the airways and make breathing more difficult, especially for asthmatics

- Carbon monoxide, which competes with oxygen for placement on red blood cells

Apply the pollution training guidelines shown in Table 4.6 in your fitness program.

Table 4.7 summarizes the CVE training principles, using the FITT acronym. Note that there is progression built into this table as you move from low to high fitness.

Suggested Readings

American College of Sports Medicine. (1992). *ACSM fitness book*. Champaign, IL: Human Kinetics.

Brown, R.L., & Henderson, J. (1994). *Fitness running*. Champaign, IL: Human Kinetics.

Burke, E.R. (1986). *Science of cycling*. Champaign, IL: Human Kinetics.

Carmichael, C., & Burke, E.R. (1994). *Fitness cycling*. Champaign, IL: Human Kinetics.

Clark, J. (1992). *Full life fitness*. Champaign, IL: Human Kinetics.

Gaines, M.P. (1993). *Fantastic water workouts*. Champaign, IL: Human Kinetics.

Gullion, L. (1993). *Nordic skiing*. Champaign, IL: Human Kinetics.

Gullion, L. (1994). *Canoeing*. Champaign, IL: Human Kinetics.

Martin, D., & Coe, P. (1991). *Training distance runners*. Champaign, IL: Human Kinetics.

Noakes, T.D. (1991). *Lore of running*. Champaign, IL: Human Kinetics.

Powell, M., & Svensson, J. (1993). *In-line skating*. Champaign, IL: Human Kinetics.

Seaborg, E. & Dudley, E. (1994). *Hiking and backpacking*. Champaign, IL: Human Kinetics.

Solis, K.M. (1992). *Ropics*. Champaign, IL: Human Kinetics.

Table 4.7
FITT Formula for Cardiovascular Endurance Training

Factor	Low fitness	Average fitness	High fitness
Frequency	3 days/week	3-5 days/week	3-7 days/week
Intensity	50%-60%	50%-70%	50%-80%
Time	20 minutes	20-60 minutes	>30 minutes
Type	Walk, swim, cycle	Previous types plus run, group exercise, row, aerobic dance	Previous types plus cross-country skiing, step aerobics

CHAPTER 5

Resistance Training for Muscular Strength and Endurance

When you hear the term *strength training*, do you picture an Arnold Schwarzenegger type lifting huge weights in the gym? For anyone who has never participated in a strength training program, that would be a likely response, and would also likely be quite intimidating. But even Arnold went into the gym for the first time one day, and he didn't get that body overnight. Not that the goal of your strength training program needs to be, or should be, that type of physique. In fact, unless you chose your parents very carefully, it probably isn't possible.

This chapter will give you the information you need to design a program to improve both your strength and muscular endurance and help improve your performance. You will also learn different ways to develop muscular strength and endurance.

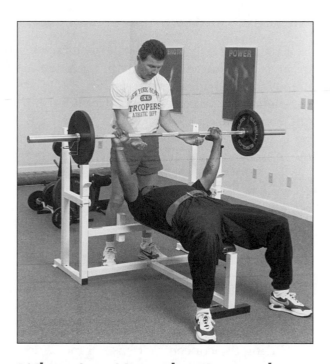

When you finish this chapter, you will be able to:

- ✪ Explain the difference between muscular strength and muscular endurance.
- ✪ Understand how the principles of training apply to resistance training.
- ✪ Develop an individual resistance training program.
- ✪ Know what activities will produce strength and endurance training effects.
- ✪ Begin a training program for this component of physical fitness.

What Are Muscular Strength and Muscular Endurance?

We all have a pretty good idea of what the term *strength* means. However, we sometimes confuse muscular strength with muscular endurance. In its purest sense, strength is the muscles' ability to generate maximum force. A muscle can overcome a given resistance through its range of motion one time. Resistance is generally some amount of weight that you are lifting or pushing, for example a set of dumbbells. However, it could be your own body weight while doing a push-up or pull-up, or the opposition presented by a partner while doing partner-resisted exercises.

Muscular endurance is the muscle's ability to overcome a given resistance for multiple repetitions or for an extended time without too much fatigue. For example, it requires a certain amount of strength in the chest, shoulders, and triceps to do a push-up. To do 30 push-ups requires the same amount of strength, but also requires some muscular endurance.

Resistance training is specific to the type of contraction that the muscle performs. Three types of contraction exist: isometric, isotonic, and isokinetic.

Isometric Contractions

Isometric contractions (or static contractions) involve the muscle contracting against an immovable and unvarying resistance. For example, standing in an open doorway and pushing out against the door jambs would be an isometric contraction. These contractions strengthen the muscle only at the angle at which the exercise is performed, not through the entire range of motion. Isometric exercises should not be done by those with cardiac conditions, as such exercises elevate blood pressure.

Isotonic Contractions

Isotonic contractions occur when the muscle goes through two phases of contraction, concentric and eccentric:

- During the concentric phase of movement the muscle shortens. Sometimes this is called positive work. Figure 5.1a shows the concentric phase as the weight is lifted in an arm curl.

- During the eccentric phase of movement the muscle lengthens back to normal. Sometimes this is called negative work. Figure 5.1b shows the eccentric phase as the weight is lowered in an arm curl.

Most resistance training programs (whether free weight, machine, or calisthenic) are isotonic training programs because you live in an isotonic world. Daily use of muscles, whether at work, play, or sports, requires isotonic contractions.

Isokinetic Contractions

Isokinetic contractions occur when the speed of contraction is controlled and the resistance accommodates to the force applied. Isokinetic contractions are only concentric. Special equipment is required to produce isokinetic contractions.

Muscle strength (force) depends on two factors:

- **Size.** The larger the cross-sectional size of the muscle, the greater the force that can be generated.

- **Fiber recruitment.** Muscles are made up of bundles of fibers. When a muscle contracts, only a percentage of the fibers contract at a single time. Consequently, the more fibers contracting, the greater the force.

Two factors that affect muscle development are gender and the type of muscle fibers present:

- **Gender.** Men tend to accommodate to resistance training by increasing size, women by increasing fiber recruitment. The reason is that men have more testosterone (a male sex hormone) than women, and testosterone builds tissue.

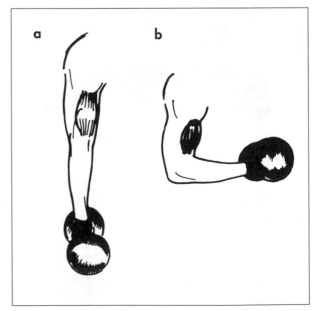

Figure 5.1 *Arm curl: (a) concentric contraction, (b) eccentric contraction.*

■ **Type of muscle fibers.** We have two basic types of muscle fibers. One type responds better to resistance training than the other does. Heredity determines how much of each fiber type we have, which explains why two people may train identically but one develops more strength. Training improves the functional ability of both types of fibers.

Law enforcement activities that require muscular strength and endurance (MSE) include:

■ Use-of-force situations

■ Climbing

■ Lifting and carrying

■ Dragging

■ Pushing

Muscular strength and endurance are related to health because they:

■ Help prevent injury

■ Delay onset of osteoporosis

■ Help prevent lower-back pain

Designing Your Program

This section will discuss the principles of training most pertinent to resistance training. These principles apply to all forms of resistance training, but weight training will be used as the example here. Officer Roberts will serve as an example for designing the program, and the answer to the questions of how often, how hard, how long, and what activities, will help her fill in the FITT chart (p. 30):

The following principles of exercise are especially important to resistance training:

■ Overload   ■ Recovery

■ Progression   ■ Balance

■ Specificity   ■ Variety

■ Regularity

Overload

For a muscle to increase strength or endurance, you must place a higher workload on the mus-

cle than is provided by your normal daily activity. Workload can be defined in terms of resistance (pounds lifted), the number of sets, and the number of repetitions in each set of repeated exercises. Over time, with regular workouts, the accumulated infinitesimal increases in muscle size become visible, and you can see musculature develop. Look at the increase in muscle size shown in Figure 5.2. As with cardiovascular endurance, overload relates to two components of FITT, intensity and time (duration).

Intensity

One of the variables in resistance training is how much weight will be lifted for each exercise. One method often used for determining intensity is to work with percentages of the most weight you can lift in one all-out effort, called one-repetition maximum (1RM). The procedure is as follows:

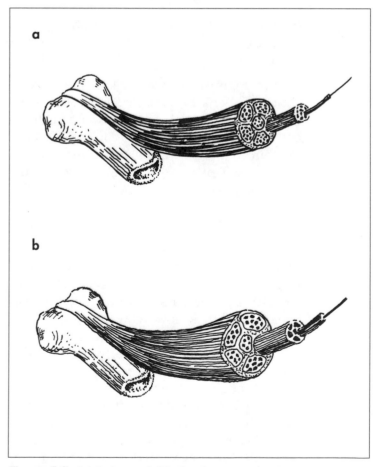

Figure 5.2 *(a) Before and (b) after long-term training, when the size of muscle fibers has increased.*

- Select exercises. Select the exercises for your program, or find ones that work on the same muscle groups. Your routine should exercise the major muscle groups necessary for basic physical movement and physical performance. These are shown in Figure 5.3.

- Determine the 1RM for each exercise. For each exercise, start with a weight that you can easily lift one time. Add weight until you have determined the most weight you can lift in one try. This is your 1RM.

Depending on whether you are trying to develop strength, endurance, or a combination of both, the percentage of the 1RM that you work with will vary from 40% to 95%.

- If the goal is muscular strength, use high resistance (80% to 95% of 1RM).

- If the goal is muscular endurance, use low resistance (40% to 60% of 1RM).

- If the goal is a combination of strength and endurance, use medium resistance (60% to 80% of 1RM).

In Figure 5.4 (see p. 42), the exercises Officer Roberts has selected are listed in the left column. Her 1RM is in the second column, and her starting weight (60% of her 1RM) is in the third. Figure 5.5 is a blank form for you to use to develop your own resistance training plan (see p. 42).

Time or Duration

While you won't actually be timing your resistance workouts as you will your CVE workouts, we will use the term "time" for consistency. The equivalent of time for resistance training is how many repetitions and sets you do of each exercise.

A repetition is the performance of an exercise from the starting position through the full range of motion and back to the start. Sets are predetermined numbers of repetitions done consecutively. New exercisers should start with one set of each exercise per workout. More advanced exercisers can start with three.

- For increasing strength, do 2 to 6 reps per set.

- For increasing endurance, do 15 to 20 reps per set.

- For increasing both strength and endurance, do 8 to 12 reps per set.

Officer Roberts wants to improve both her strength and her endurance. If you share that desire, here is how to determine the starting weights for your program:

- Determine 60% to 80% of the 1RM for each exercise. Start with 60% of your 1RM and see if you can do eight reps correctly. If not, reduce the weight until you can. If you can do 12 reps correctly, increase the weight until you reach a weight for which 8 to 11 reps can be done correctly before reaching muscle failure—when you can no longer perform a correct repetition of the exercise. Use that weight until you can do 12 reps correctly. For sit-ups and trunk lifts (back extensions), divide the number done in 1 minute by one-half for the number of training repetitions.

Officer Roberts will start with one set of each exercise. To build both strength and endurance, she should do 8 to 12 reps per set.

Progression

As a muscle adjusts to the new workload, the workload must be increased again to continue improvement. Increase resistance when 12 reps are reached. For each exercise, increase the weight by 5 to 10% once 12 reps can be done correctly. Between 8 and 11 reps should be possible with the new weight. For the sit-ups and trunk lifts, retest every 4 weeks.

Gradually work up to and maintain three sets of the exercises for each training session. If you have the time and motivation, do up to five sets.

Officer Roberts is planning to train 3 days per week, starting with 60% of her 1RM, and doing one set of 8 to 12 reps. As her conditioning improves, she may decide to alter parts of her training plan. She may find that

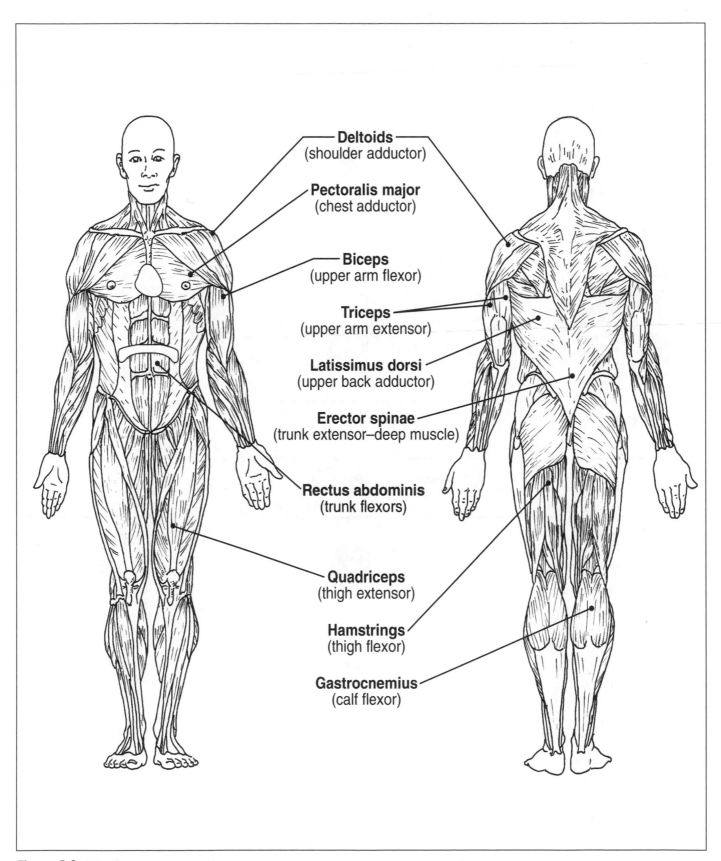

Deltoids
(shoulder adductor)

Pectoralis major
(chest adductor)

Biceps
(upper arm flexor)

Triceps
(upper arm extensor)

Latissimus dorsi
(upper back adductor)

Erector spinae
(trunk extensor–deep muscle)

Rectus abdominis
(trunk flexors)

Quadriceps
(thigh extensor)

Hamstrings
(thigh flexor)

Gastrocnemius
(calf flexor)

Figure 5.3 *Muscle groups to exercise.*

Exercise	1RM	Beginning weight	Week 1 sets (8-12 reps)	Week 2 sets (8-12 reps)	Week 3 sets (8-12 reps)	Week 4 sets (8-12 reps)
Leg press/ squat	130	80	1	2	3	3
Bench press	40	25	1	2	3	3
Leg flexion	40	25	1	2	3	3
Bent rowing/ pull-down	50	30	1	2	3	3
Military/ shoulder press	60	35	1	2	3	3
Sit-ups/ abdominal curls	28	14	1	2	3	3
Trunk lifts/ back extension	12	6	1	2	3	3
Calf raises	180	100	1	2	3	3
Biceps curls	30	20	1	2	3	3
Triceps extension	30	20	1	2	3	3

Figure 5.4 *Resistance training plan for Officer Roberts.*

Exercise	1RM	Beginning weight	Week 1 sets (8-12 reps)	Week 2 sets (8-12 reps)	Week 3 sets (8-12 reps)	Week 4 sets (8-12 reps)
Leg press/ squat	_____	_____	_____	_____	_____	_____
Bench press	_____	_____	_____	_____	_____	_____
Leg flexion	_____	_____	_____	_____	_____	_____
Bent rowing/ pull-down	_____	_____	_____	_____	_____	_____
Military/ shoulder press	_____	_____	_____	_____	_____	_____
Sit-ups/ abdominal curls	_____	_____	_____	_____	_____	_____
Trunk lifts/ back extension	_____	_____	_____	_____	_____	_____
Calf raises	_____	_____	_____	_____	_____	_____
Biceps curls	_____	_____	_____	_____	_____	_____
Triceps extension	_____	_____	_____	_____	_____	_____

Figure 5.5 *Resistance training planning form.*

her schedule precludes training any more often than three times per week, but that she can complete the workout with a higher percentage of her 1RM. She should also gradually increase the number of sets until she reaches three. As she increases the number of sets, she may have to cut back on the amount of weight she is lifting, especially in the last set. That's OK because as her muscles adapt to the new overload she will be able to eventually get to where she can complete three sets with the heavier weight.

Specificity

Training is specific to the muscle, the contraction movement, the joint angle, the apparatus or equipment used, and the demand placed on the muscle. Upper body training will not increase lower body strength, and vice versa. Select a series of exercises to work a wide range of muscle groups.

Regularity

Resistance training must be consistent over time. Strength cannot be saved up; it must be maintained constantly with regular resistance training. Recent evidence indicates that strength gains may take place with as few as two training sessions per week. More fit people may choose to train more often.

Recovery

Although regular exercise is crucial, the same muscle should not be worked to exhaustion on consecutive days. The muscle needs time to recover before being worked again. To apply this principle to resistance training, consider the following guidelines:

- Those just beginning a training program should alternate days of training with days of rest.

- More advanced exercisers may train on consecutive days but avoid working the same muscle group on two consecutive days. Two examples of how more advanced exercisers may apply the principle of recovery are shown in Table 5.1.

Table 5.1 Sample Resistance Training Schedules for More Advanced Exercisers	
Alternate days	**Alternate body parts**
Sunday— Rest	Sunday— Rest
Monday— All body parts	Monday— Upper body
Tuesday— Rest	Tuesday— Lower body
Wednesday— All body parts	Wednesday— Rest
Thursday—Rest Rest	Thursday— Upper body
Friday— All body parts	Friday— Lower body
Saturday— Rest	Saturday— Rest

You should also consider scheduling days of rest before and after your agency's fitness test, or before and after any all-out effort.

Based on her assessment, Officer Roberts' muscular fitness is average. Because she has not been working out on a regular basis, she will begin by training every other day.

Balance

Because of specificity, all muscles should be exercised regularly to avoid an imbalance between muscles and to develop overall body strength and endurance. Muscular strength imbalances can cause injuries. Resistance training can be applied to all muscles that provide movement. Very specific routines can be developed to increase muscle strength and performance in particular ways.

Table 5.2 shows the muscle groups and the free weight and exercise machine exercises that work them. The free weight exercises are described in detail in Appendix A. Many different types of machines are available for each exercise. Although they are similar, it is important to refer to the instructional manual for each machine to ensure proper execution.

Table 5.2
Weight Training Exercises

Muscle group	Free weights	Exercise machines	Recommendations and cautions
Gastrocnemius	Heel raises with weight on back	Calf raises	Use a 2″ lift. Do 10 reps with toes pointed straight ahead, 10 pointed out, and 10 pointed in.
Quadriceps	Half-knee bends (or squats) with weight on back	Leg press or leg extensions	For free weights, lower buttocks until thigh is parallel to ground. Keep movements smooth without any bouncing.
Hamstrings	Leg flexion	Leg flexion	Resistance should be enough that it takes 2 seconds to raise the leg, 4 seconds to lower it.
Abdominals	Sit-ups	Abdominal curl machine	For sit-ups, keep legs bent at 90° angle. Don't lift buttocks off the ground.
Erector spinae	Trunk lifts	Back extension machine	Not recommended for those with back problems.
Pectorals	Bench press	Bench press	Do not arch back.
Latissimus dorsi	Bent rowing	Pull down	Pull bar to chest, not stomach.
Deltoids	Military press	Seated shoulder press	For free weights, alternate lowering weight in front of and behind head. Keep back straight.
Biceps	Curls	Curls	
Triceps	Triceps extension	Triceps extension	With free weights, this exercise also can be done lying on a bench.

If you do not have access to the manual, get some instruction and supervision from a more experienced person.

Variety

As with any training, doing the same routine over and over again will get boring. You can attain a strength and endurance training effect in any number of ways. As you become more experienced, look for new exercises to train the same muscle groups. If you have access to several different types of equipment, try them. For a change of pace, consider occasionally doing the calisthenic routine described later in this chapter.

Using free weights or machines, or even pushing against the resistance of a partner, can help you achieve the desired effect.

Officer Roberts has access to a Universal multistation machine in her agency's fitness room, and plans to use it for her workouts.

Officer Roberts' completed individual resistance training plan is shown here.

Frequency _____	3 times per week
Intensity _____	60–80% of 1RM
Time _____	One set of 8–12 reps
Type _____	Universal machine

Additional Strength Training Tips

There are a number of lessons not covered by the principles of exercise that will make your training safer and more effective.

1. Warm up with calisthenics and stretching for 3 to 5 minutes before doing a resistance workout. Part of the warm-up can be lifting lighter weights than what you normally train with.

2. Start with the largest muscle groups and work down to the smallest. Small muscles are generally involved at least as stabilizers when you exercise the larger muscles. If you exhaust them before you complete training the larger muscles, you will be unable to get as much work done with the larger muscles. If you plan to exercise all the major muscle groups in the same workout, a recommended sequence would be legs, back, chest, shoulders, arms, and neck. The abdominals can be exercised every day if you desire.

3. Exercise the muscles through the full range of motion (FROM). Before performing an exercise for the first time, simulate the movement of the body part to be exercised as far as it can go from the starting position to full extension and back again. This is the full range of motion of that muscle for that exercise. Start from the stretched position, move to the contracted position, and then return to the stretched position. For maximum strength gains, it is important to do each exercise through the FROM.

4. Control the weight, and avoid fast and jerky movements. The purpose of this rule is to avoid injury while getting the maximum benefit out of each repetition. Lift the weight with a smooth, controlled motion. Do not "throw" the weight. Counting to two as you lift the weight will give you about the right speed of movement. Lower the weight slowly, counting to four because the negative phase should take about twice as long as the positive phase.

There are reasons for this. First, the same muscles are used to lower the weight as to lift it. Second, you can lower much more weight than you can lift, so there is potential for more strength gain in the negative phase. If you are working with a partner, include some negative work in each session. Have your partner help you lift a weight that you can't lift by yourself, and then slowly lower it. Repeat until you can no longer safely control the weight's descent. Or at the end of a regular set of an exercise, when you can no longer lift a weight by yourself, have your partner help

you back to the starting position and then you lower the weight. Repeat until you can no longer safely control its descent.

5. Exercise a muscle to momentary failure. A muscle consists of thousands of individual fibers. For each bout of work, only as many fibers as are required to accomplish the work are "recruited" for the job. To ensure maximum participation of the fibers, it is necessary to work the muscle to exhaustion.

6. Rest between each set of exercises: for endurance, 1.5 to 2 minutes; for strength, 3 to 5 minutes; for both, 30 to 60 seconds.

7. Practice proper form. For most people it is more comfortable to exhale while lifting the weight and inhale while lowering the weight. Do not hold your breath or hyperventilate. If training with free weights, keep the weights close to the body.

8. Whenever possible, work with a partner. There are three advantages to this. One is that you are more likely to push yourself when someone is there with you. Another is that you can more easily accomplish negative work. Finally, it is safer to work with a partner.

You and your partner should know how to "spot" for each other. Spotters are essential for free-weight lifters. They provide the following benefits:

- Ensure that weights don't fall on the lifter or others
- Give the lifter confidence to try heavier weights or do additional repetitions
- Offer motivation
- Assist the lifter as he or she reaches muscular failure

Spotters should have the following qualities:

- Enough strength to assist with the weights being lifted
- Knowledge about where to stand and how to grip the bar
- Alertness for signs of trouble

Table 5.3		
Calisthenic Exercises		
Muscle group	**Calisthenic exercise**	**Description**
Gastrocnemius	Heel raise	Hands on hips, rise up on toes as high as possible. Increase range of motion by placing toes on 2-inch board.
Quadriceps	Half-knee bends	Feet shoulder-width apart, back straight, hands on hips, squat until thighs are parallel to ground, and return to start.
Hamstrings	Assisted leg curl	Lie face down, curl one leg toward buttocks, partner resisting. Resist partner as he or she pulls leg to start position.**
Abdominals	Sit-up with arms crossed*	Start on back, knees bent 90°, arms crossed on chest. Sit up, touch elbows to knees, and return.**
Erector spinae	Trunk lifts*	Lie on stomach, hands flat on floor, elbows bent. Raise trunk off floor.**
Pectorals and deltoids	Push-ups	Toes on ground, hands on ground shoulder-width apart. Keep back straight. Lower upper body to ground, and return to start.
Latissimus dorsi	Bent rowing (Use books or other weighted objects)	Bend forward at waist, lower object in each hand until arms outstretched, return.
Biceps	Chin-ups or flexed-arm hangs	Hang from bar with arms straight, pull up until chin is above bar, return to hanging position.
Triceps	Chair dips	Back to chair. Grasp sides of stable chair, feet straight in front. Lower body as far as possible and push back up.

*These exercises are contraindicated for those who have back problems.
**See descriptions in Appendix A.

- Willingness to encourage the lifter to make a maximum effort and to maintain correct form

For spotting to work, the lifter must communicate with the spotter. The lifter must tell the spotter how many reps he or she plans to attempt and during what rep he or she is likely to need help.

Developing a Calisthenic Training Plan

Some officers may not be strong enough to begin a resistance training program using weights or machines. For these officers, their body weight may provide sufficient overload. Others may not have access to equipment. For these officers, anything will be better than nothing. And every officer will at one time or another be without equipment, for example when traveling. In these situations, consider using calisthenics as your resistance training activity.

Calisthenic training employs exercises in which one's body weight and gravity supply the resistance. Calisthenic routines work very well for developing muscular endurance, but they provide only minimal muscular strength development (unless the individual has low strength). In a calisthenic routine, the individual usually performs three sets of exercises and gradually increases repetitions over time. Table 5.3 lists calisthenics and the muscle groups that they exercise.

In the calisthenic training program, perform each set as a circuit. In other words, do one set of each exercise in sequence, then start again with the first exercise and proceed through the sequence for the second set, then again for the third set.

To develop a calisthenic training plan, follow this sequence:

1. Select exercises. Choose the exercises listed above, or find ones that work on the same muscle groups.

2. Determine the number of repetitions. Test yourself to see how many repetitions of each exercise you can do in 1 minute.

3. Sequence the exercises. Follow the principle of moving from large muscle groups to small ones, and alternate the muscle groups. (This is done on the form for you.)

4. Start the program. Do one set of repetitions of each exercise, i.e., the number of repetitions done in 1 minute.

5. Change at Week 2. Divide the number of repetitions for each exercise by one half and add a second set. Each set will have half the repetitions done in the first week.

6. Change again at Week 3. Add a third set of repetitions, again half of the repetitions done in the first week.

7. Maintain. Stay at three sets, but add one to two repetitions each week to each set of each exercise.

Use Figure 5.6 to outline a calisthenic training plan.

Exercise	1 minute reps	1/2 reps	Week 1 rep/sets	Week 2 rep/sets	Week 3 rep/sets	Week 4 rep/sets
Half-knee bends	____	____	____	____	____	____
Push-ups	____	____	____	____	____	____
Assisted leg curls	____	____	____	____	____	____
Bent rowing	____	____	____	____	____	____
Sit-ups	____	____	____	____	____	____
Trunk lifts	____	____	____	____	____	____
Calf raises	____	____	____	____	____	____
Chin-ups/ flexed-arm hang	____	____	____	____	____	____
Chair dips	____	____	____	____	____	____

Figure 5.6 *Calisthenic training plan.*

Table 5.4 summarizes the information you need to design your resistance training plan, using the FITT acronym:

Table 5.4 Summary of Resistance Training Principles			
	FITNESS LEVEL		
Factor	**Low**	**Average**	**High**
Frequency	3 days/week	3-4 days/week	4-6 days/week
Intensity			
Endurance	40%	40-50%	40-60%
Strength	80%	80-90%	80-95%
Both	60%	60-70%	60-80%
Time	1 set	3 sets	3-5 sets
Endurance (1.5 minutes rest between sets)	15-20 reps	15-20 reps	15-20 reps
Strength (3-5 minutes rest between sets)	2-6 reps	2-6 reps	2-6 reps
Both (30-60 seconds rest between sets)	8-12 reps	8-12 reps	8-12 reps
Type	Calisthenics, machines	Calisthenics, free weights, machines	Free weights, machines

Suggested Readings

Baechle, T.R. (Ed.) (1994). *Essentials of strength training and conditioning*. Champaign, IL: Human Kinetics.

Baechle, T.R., & Groves, B.R. (1992). *Weight training: Steps to success*. Champaign, IL: Human Kinetics.

Baechle, T.R., & Groves, B.R. (1994). *Weight training instruction: Steps to success*. Champaign, IL: Human Kinetics.

Fleck, S.J., & Kraemer, W.J. (1987). *Designing resistance training programs*. Champaign, IL: Human Kinetics.

Komi, P.V. (Ed.) (1992). *Strength and power in sport: The encyclopedia of sports medicine*. Champaign, IL: Human Kinetics.

Kubistant, T. (1988). *Mind pump*. Champaign, IL: Human Kinetics.

Peterson, J.A. (Ed.) (1982). *Total fitness: The Nautilus way* (2nd ed.). Champaign, IL: Human Kinetics.

Riley, D.P. (Ed.) (1982). *Strength training by the experts* (2nd ed.). Champaign, IL: Human Kinetics.

CHAPTER 6

Flexibility

How many times have you felt "tight" when starting a physical activity? Do you remember your youth coaches telling you to "bounce it out, make it hurt" when you were warming up for a game or practice? How many times have you started out a run feeling sore and told yourself that the run would work the soreness out? Do your muscles often feel stiff when you get out of your patrol car?

This chapter will teach you how to change each of these experiences. You will learn that not only is it important to stretch regularly, but it is important to stretch correctly. You will also learn that there are two primary purposes of stretching: to avoid injury and to improve flexibility.

What Is Flexibility?

Flexibility is the range of motion of part of the body. All other things being equal, the more

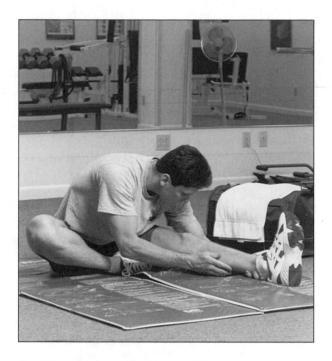

flexible you are, the better able you are to perform a given physical function.

When you stretch an area of the body, the tough connective tissue covering the muscle, as well as the muscle itself, is heated up and becomes more pliable. As a result, the muscle responds better to subsequent movement and is better prepared for more rigorous activity which may follow.

For a simple analogy, think of the muscle as a rubber band. Before you continue reading, try this experiment with a couple of rubber bands. Rapidly stretch one of them as far as you can, note how long it is, and then allow it to snap back to its original length. Now stretch it three or four more times. Notice that it's a little easier to pull each time than it was

> ### When you finish this chapter, you will be able to:
>
> - ✪ Explain what flexibility is, and understand why it is important for law enforcement officers.
> - ✪ Understand how the principles of exercise apply to flexibility training.
> - ✪ Develop a flexibility training program.
> - ✪ Begin a training program for this component of physical fitness.

at first. You can also stretch it further on each subsequent pull. That's because it has actually "warmed up" as you've pulled on it.

Now take the other rubber band and stretch it slowly. Because it is being pulled slowly, even on the first pull it will stretch more than the one you stretched rapidly. This is how your muscles respond. Rapid, jerky movements before they are warmed up can hurt them. Slow, gradual stretching produces better results.

Law enforcement activities that require flexibility include:

- Vehicle dismount

- Emergency extraction

- Any activity requiring bending and reaching

Flexibility is related to injury prevention because it:

- Reduces the chance of injury when suddenly going from inactivity to rapid movement

- Helps lower the incidence of lower-back pain

Designing Your Program

The principles of exercise also apply to flexibility training. As you learned in the last two chapters, the key questions to be answered in designing fitness programs are:

- How often?

- How hard?

- How long?

- What activity?

Once again, the FITT chart (p. 30) will be used to record the answer to each of the key questions. For this component of fitness, we will use Officer Johnson as our example.

The principles of exercise most applicable to flexibility training are:

- Individuality
- Overload
- Progression
- Specificity
- Regularity
- Recovery
- Balance
- Variety

Individuality

As you learned in chapter 3, each of you will respond differently to the same training routine. This is particularly true for flexibility. Age, gender, and previous training are contributors to these differences. The key point to remember is that stretching is not a contest, and you need to train within your limitations. Take a simple exercise like bending at the waist with the objective of touching your toes. In a group of four people doing this exercise, you might find one who can put her or his palms flat on the ground, while another touches the toes, and the third gets to the ankles. If you can only reach your knees, you may feel a little embarrassed. Your competitiveness may cause you to try and match the others in the group. You may start bouncing in an effort to add a few inches to your stretch. Or you may bend your knees, or "cheat" in some other way. As you will learn later in this chapter, neither solution is helpful.

The point of this example is that you have to take your individuality into account when you are doing your stretching. You needn't be concerned with how much further they can stretch than you can. While you may never become as limber as an Olympic gymnast, your flexibility will improve with regular stretching.

Overload

To get a training effect, you must stretch the muscles beyond where daily activities take them. If your typical day includes getting out of bed, getting in and out of your car 10 to 20 times, walking, sitting, and then getting back into bed, you won't have to do much to exceed those demands.

Overload affects two components of FITT, intensity and time. They are defined by how hard you should stretch the muscles, and how long you should hold each stretch.

Intensity

Let's try an activity that will show you how hard to stretch. While standing, bend forward at the waist, and let your arms hang in front of you. You should feel the muscles in the back of the legs stretching. Hold that position for a count of 10, note how far you were able to reach, and return to the upright position. The slight pressure you felt on the backs of your legs is how intense stretching should feel. You should feel slight discomfort but not pain. If it hurts, then you need to back off.

Try the same stretch again, and again note how far you have reached. Before returning to the upright position, grab the backs of your legs and gently pull your head toward your legs. You will feel additional pressure, and possibly even pain. That is the point where you need to back off.

Time

The length of time you hold a stretch will differ depending upon the purpose of your program. When stretching as part of your warm-up and cool-down, hold each stretch for 10 to 20 seconds. Repeat each exercise three times, or until the muscle feels loose.

When stretching to improve flexibility, you should hold the stretches for 30 to 60 seconds, and do 5 to 10 repetitions of each.

Progression

This principle can be applied both to individual workouts and to the overall program. When you tried to touch your toes earlier, you probably found that you came closer on your second attempt than you did on the first. If you had tried a third time, you would have stretched a little further yet. Within each workout, as the muscle warms and becomes more pliable, you will find that you can stretch it more, up to the point of your current maximum flexibility.

It may also help to start with easier stretches and progress to the more difficult ones. For example, seated stretches are less taxing than standing ones.

Over time, you will be able to continue to improve your point of maximum flexibility. Eventually you may reach a point where you can no longer improve without assistance. At that point you may consider using partner-assisted stretches.

Specificity

Flexibility training is specific to the muscles being stretched. Stretching the hamstrings will do nothing for the shoulders, and vice versa. Therefore, it is important to concentrate your warm-up on the muscles to be used during the exercises that follow. While doing your strength training, you may want to stretch the appropriate muscles during rest periods between sets. During your cool-down, again focus on the muscles used in the preceding exercise activity. For example, if you were doing strength training for the upper body, stretch the chest, arms, back, shoulders, and torso after the workout. Also, as you become more familiar with your body, give extra attention to the areas that are sore and require a little more effort to get loose.

Specificity also applies to the type of stretch used. The three main types are ballistic, static, and partner-assisted.

Ballistic Stretching

When your youth coach told you to "bounce it out, make it hurt," you were doing ballistic stretches. Ballistic stretching involves rapid, jerky movements, and shouldn't be done at full speed until the muscles have been warmed up and stretched with static stretches. Then you might use them as a bridge from the warm-up to the more rigorous activity to follow. If they hurt, you probably aren't warmed up enough.

Your well-intentioned but possibly ill-informed youth coaches may have used ballistic stretches exactly opposite to the way they should have been used. If it weren't for the fact that you were young and resilient, they might have done considerable damage to your body. Try to imagine what that might feel like today!

Ballistic stretches include any movement in which the muscle moves through a range of motion rapidly and then bounces back to the starting position. Many of the static stretches you will learn later can be done as ballistic stretches if so desired.

Static Stretching

The preferred exercises for warming up, cooling down, and improving our flexibility are static stretches. Static stretching involves using body weight to slowly stretch the muscle. There should not be any pain involved, and you should stretch the muscle only to the point of slight discomfort. Rather than bouncing, the stretch should be a slow, smooth movement, and you should continue breathing normally throughout the exercise. Stretch both at the beginning of an exercise session to prepare the muscles for the more rigorous activity to follow, and at the end to reduce soreness.

Partner-Assisted Stretching

A third type of stretching is partner-assisted. These stretches are more advanced and involve having a partner gently help you to stretch beyond a point you can reach by yourself. Be aware that there is high potential for injury if the partner is unfamiliar with the technique or you fail to communicate with each other.

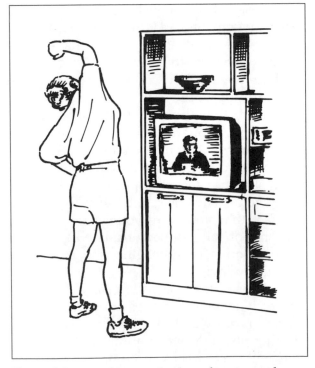

Figure 6.1 *Stretching can be done almost anywhere.*

Regularity

Use it or lose it. As with the other components of physical fitness, regularity is essential. At a minimum you should do some stretching before and after every exercise session. These warm-up and cool-down periods, as you will learn later in this chapter, help prevent injury and reduce soreness. They will also help improve your flexibility. But to seriously change your flexibility, you should plan some additional training that concentrates solely on stretching. Even as busy as your days are, you should be able to find time for some stretching. For example, you might spend a minute or two stretching each time you get out of your patrol car. (See Appendix B for some sample stretches to do for your back, hips, and shoulders.)

Recovery

Unlike the other components of fitness, there is no need for recovery between workouts. You can stretch every day, and in fact this is a good habit to develop. Stretching can be relaxing, you can do it anywhere, and it doesn't necessitate working up a sweat. You can do it in your work area periodically throughout the day, or in front of the TV at night (see Figure 6.1). Adding these extra sessions to your program can have a significant impact on improving your flexibility.

After learning about the application of the principles of regularity and recovery, Officer Johnson decides to incorporate daily flexibility sessions into his training plan. In addition to his warm-up and cool-down sessions, he is going to spend 30 minutes each day stretching to improve his overall flexibility.

Balance

Your plan should include all areas of the body. These areas may vary from workout to workout, but over time your plan should include all of the ones listed in Figure 6.2.

When planning your warm-up, cool-down, and flexibility improvement, select the body parts to be stretched, and choose appropriate stretches from Appendix B. As a minimum, do the stretches in Figure 6.3. If you know of other stretches, use them too.

Variety

In Appendix B, we'll show some sample stretches for each major muscle group. There are hundreds of others, and as you experiment with your flexibility program you will discover others that may work better for you. Also consider changing your routine from time to time to avoid boredom. You can find additional stretches, including sport-specific stretches, in *Sport Stretch* by Michael J. Alter.

Officer Johnson now has the last bit of information he needs to complete his flexibility training plan.

Frequency _____Before and after each CVE and MSE workout. Daily flexibility improvement sessions for 30 minutes during the evening news.

Intensity ___Stretch to the point of discomfort, not pain.

Time_____10–20 seconds during warm-up/cool-down; 30–60 seconds during flexibility development.

Type ____One minute of easy jogging in place to warm the muscles. Three repetitions of selected static stretches as part of warm-up and cool-down. Five repetitions of the selected static stretches for improved flexibility.

Ankles	Abdominals	Lower leg
Lower back	Achilles tendon	Trunk
Back of knee	Upper back	Hamstrings
Neck	Quadriceps	Pectorals
Groin	Shoulders	Hip flexors
Biceps	Buttocks	Triceps

Figure 6.2 *Body areas to stretch.*

Lower leg, p. 115	Lower back, p. 118
Achilles tendon, p. 116	Trunk, p. 119
Shoulders, p. 120	Upper back, p. 119
Hamstrings, p. 116	Biceps, p. 121
Quadriceps, p. 117	Triceps, p. 121

Figure 6.3 *Minimum static stretching exercises.*

Additional Flexibility Training Tips

To make your training safer and more effective, follow these tips:

1. The elasticity of the muscles diminishes with age and inactivity. Consider these factors if you are just beginning an exercise regimen. Go slowly, and be prepared for some muscle soreness.

2. When you train, follow these guidelines:

   ■ Warm the muscles with some easy jogging in place or jumping jacks.

   ■ Start with the easier exercises and progress to the harder ones. Seated exercises, for example, generally are less stressful than standing ones and thus should be done first. It is also more convenient to do all the seated ones while you are on the ground.

   ■ Stretch the muscle through the full range of motion, letting your body weight do the work. For instance, when you try to touch your toes, lean forward at the waist and let gravity pull you down.

3. Don't stretch the affected area under the following conditions:

   ■ You've had a recent fracture of a bone

   ■ You have sharp, acute pain with joint movement or muscle elongation

   ■ You've had a recent sprain or strain

4. It is better to do the stretch correctly, even if you can't reach as far as the picture shows, than to "cheat." In time you'll see more improvement if you do the stretches properly than if you are doing them incorrectly.

Warm-Up and Cool-Down

We have made several references to warm-up and cool-down. While by now you may have a pretty good idea of what they entail, here's a brief description of what they are and how they are accomplished.

Warm up before physical activity to prepare the muscles for the more vigorous activity to follow. Warming up provides a transition as the body moves from rest to activity. It helps prevent injury and enhances performance. The warm-up has two parts: light movement, followed by static stretches. Start with some easy, rhythmic movements to warm the muscle. A good rule of thumb is to do enough easy running in place or jumping jacks to develop a light sweat prior to stretching. The static stretching part of the warm-up should concentrate on the muscles to be used in the activity to follow.

Many people who wouldn't think about exercising without warming up first completely ignore the cool-down. Yet easy movement and static stretching at the end of a workout may be just as important as warming up. One benefit of cooling down seems to be reduced muscle soreness. And just as the warm-up serves as a transition from rest to activity, so does the cool-down provide a gradual transition back to rest.

Table 6.1 summarizes the flexibility training principles using FITT.

Table 6.1
Principles of the Flexibility Training Plan

F—**F**requency: Flexibility training can be done every day. As a minimum, do it before and after every workout.

I—**I**ntensity: Stretch to the point of discomfort, not pain.

T—**T**ime: 10-20 seconds during warm-up/cool-down; 30-60 seconds during flexibility development.

T—**T**ype: Static stretches are preferred.

Suggested Readings

Alter, M.J. (1990). *Sport stretch*. Champaign, IL: Human Kinetics.

Anderson, B. (1980). *Stretching*. Bolinas, CA: Shelter Publications.

McAtee, R.E. (1993). *Facilitated stretching*. Champaign, IL: Human Kinetics.

CHAPTER 7

Anaerobic Fitness

Maybe you have been participating in a cardiovascular training program for some time, and routinely run distances of several miles. Yet when you run up two flights of stairs, or sprint to first base in a softball game, you find yourself breathing hard. Does it confuse you that running hard for short distances has this effect when you can run for miles and maintain a more relaxed breathing pattern?

The reason there is a difference is that you are using two different energy systems for the activities. As you learned in chapter 4, your cardiovascular system combines oxygen from the air you breathe with foodstuffs stored in your body to produce the energy necessary for the activity. However, this energy system doesn't have time to kick in for

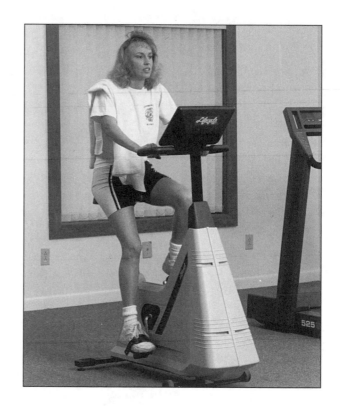

activities requiring short, intense bursts of maximal effort. That is where the anaerobic system comes into play.

What Is Anaerobic Fitness?

Anaerobic activities are those that are done in the absence of oxygen. That is, they use energy sources that are already present in the muscle. This source of energy is limited, and so anaerobic activities are of relatively short duration. For example, sprinting, pushing or pulling an object a short distance, or lifting something one time would require anaerobic energy production (see Figure 7.1).

When you finish this chapter, you will be able to:

- ✪ Explain what anaerobic fitness is, and give examples of what types of activities require it.

- ✪ Understand how the principles of exercise apply to anaerobic fitness training.

- ✪ Develop an individual anaerobic fitness training program.

- ✪ Know what activities you can participate in to improve anaerobic fitness.

- ✪ Begin a training program for this component of fitness.

Law enforcement activities that require anaerobic power include:

- Running up stairs
- Defensive tactics
- Lifting and carrying for short distances
- Pushing and pulling for short distances

There are no health benefits clearly associated with anaerobic power.

Designing Your Program

Once again you will use the principles of fitness to learn how to develop your anaerobic fitness plan. Officer Hernandez will serve as an example, and the FITT chart (p. 30) will contain the details of the program.

The principles of fitness most applicable to anaerobic training are:

- Overload
- Regularity
- Progression
- Recovery
- Specificity

Overload

To improve the anaerobic system, your training activities must be done at a faster pace than you would normally use for the activity. For example, if you are cycling, your anaerobic training would be short sprints done at a faster speed than your long rides.

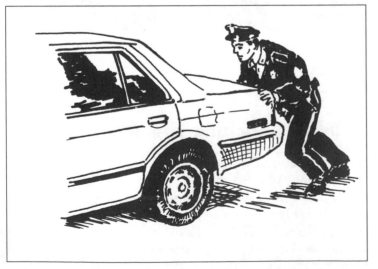

Figure 7.1 *Pushing heavy objects requires anaerobic energy production.*

Intensity

Because there is danger of injury from this more intense training, when you start out your intensity should merely exceed the speed of your cardiovascular endurance workouts. This would be about half of your all-out sprint speed.

Time

There are four variables to consider in this part of the plan:

- The distance to cover
- How fast to cover the distance
- How many repetitions to do
- How much rest to take between each repetition

If you have access to a running track, you can use it to run known distances such as 110, 220, and 440 yards. It isn't a requirement to cover known distances, but it does make charting your progress easier. Instead of a known distance you can also run for a certain period of time. For example, you might decide to run fast for 30 seconds.

Deciding on the speed of each repetition may require some experimentation. Being careful to avoid injury, start by running at a speed that is at least faster than your pace for longer distances. Time yourself on each repetition so that you have a yardstick for planning future workouts.

The number of repetitions will depend to some degree upon the distance covered. For example, if your training distance is 110 yards, you might decide to do 15 repetitions. But if you increase the distance for your repetitions to 440 yards, you could cut back the number of repetitions to four to eight. When starting out, plan for a total distance of about 1 mile of work. For example, 15 repetitions of 110 yards or 4 repetitions of 440 yards. As your conditioning improves, gradually increase the total distance to 2 miles.

The last consideration is the rest period between repetitions. As a general rule, rest for two or three times as long as the work interval is. That means if you are running 220 yards in

45 seconds, you should rest 90 to 135 seconds between runs. The rest should consist of walking or jogging, not sitting or standing still.

Progression

Over time, gradually increase the speed of your workouts until you reach about 90% of your maximal heart rate. You may also decide to increase the distance of your repetitions, increase the number of repetitions, or decrease the length of the rest period.

Officer Hernandez will start his anaerobic training program by running 10 repetitions of 60 yards, slightly faster than his regular running pace. Over the next few weeks he will increase the number of repetitions and increase the distance and the speed. After 6 weeks he will evaluate his condition and consider increasing the distance of his runs to 220 yards.

Specificity

To train the anaerobic system to improve its efficiency, use activities similar to what you are training for. If your training includes other activities, for example biking or swimming, you can use those activities for your anaerobic training. If you are primarily concerned with the 300-meter run on your agency's fitness test, as is Officer Hernandez, your best bet is to train with sprint running.

Regularity

The anaerobic system does not require as much training as the aerobic system does. With as few as one training session per week you will see eventual improvements. But regularity is important. Training less than once a week won't improve the system. Also, you will lose some of your adaptation to this type of training if it's not done regularly.

Recovery

Think back to the last time you sprinted all-out, or ran up stairs as fast as you could. Were your legs sore after the effort? How about the next day? Even when you are used to such activity it is common to have soreness afterward. The soreness is due in large part to the strain you are putting on your legs. Because this training is so hard on your body, you need a longer recovery period between exercise sessions. The potential for injury greatly outweighs the benefits of any more than two anaerobic workouts per week.

Officer Hernandez clearly needs some anaerobic conditioning since he could not finish the 300-meter run on his agency's fitness test. Because of his generally poor level of conditioning, he should limit his anaerobic training at first to one session per week.

Officer Hernandez's completed chart looks like this:

Frequency _____ One workout per week

Intensity _____ Just faster than his running speed for the 1.5-mile run

Time _____ 10 repetitions of 60 yards, with 1 minute rest between each

Type _____ Sprint training

Developing the Anaerobic Training Plan

To complete the anaerobic training plan, take these four steps:

1. Select the activity. This could be sprinting, stair climbing, bounding, swimming, or cycling.

2. Define the work interval. The work interval includes the training distance, training time for the distance, and the number of times the training distance is run.

3. Define the rest interval. This is determining the amount of time spent walking or jogging slowly between repetitions.

4. Define the frequency. This is setting the number of days on which training is done.

Training for the 300-Meter Run

In addition to wanting to improve your job performance, some of you will want to improve your time on the 300-meter run. Here is an anaerobic training program specifically designed to meet that goal. It is intended for those who have been doing some previous anaerobic training. Others should train for 8 to 10 weeks before beginning this program.

Training distance = 110-220 yds

Training time = Time an all-out effort, then start training at 80% of that time.

For example, if the all-out effort is 20 seconds, divide 20 by .80 to get your starting training time of 25 seconds.

Repetitions = 10-15

Rest time = 1-2 min

Frequency = 1 or 2 times per week

Progress to higher levels by increasing distance and repetitions and by decreasing training time.

This is how Officer Hernandez developed his anaerobic training plan.

Training distance	Repetitions	Training time	Rest	Frequency	Week
60 yards	10	12 seconds	2 minutes	1 day/week	1, 2
110 yards	12	20 seconds	2 minutes	1 day/week	3, 4
110 yards	15	17 seconds	2 minutes	1 day/week	5, 6
220 yards	8	42 seconds	2 minutes	1 day/week	7, 8
220 yards	10	40 seconds	2 minutes	1 day/week	9, 10

Figure 7.2 is a blank form you can use to develop your own anaerobic training plan:

Training distance	Repetitions	Training time	Rest	Frequency	Week
_____	_____	_____	_____	_____	_____
_____	_____	_____	_____	_____	_____
_____	_____	_____	_____	_____	_____
_____	_____	_____	_____	_____	_____
_____	_____	_____	_____	_____	_____
_____	_____	_____	_____	_____	_____

Figure 7.2 *Anaerobic training plan form.*

Additional Training Tips

These additional tips are intended to make your training safer and more effective.

1. When doing anaerobic work, you should take special precautions to avoid injury. It is important to thoroughly warm the muscles before the workout. This can be accomplished by doing some easy jogging or running in place until a light sweat forms. As a minimum, two or three repetitions of all the lower body stretches from Appendix B must be done.

2. Sprinting should start with short distances of 40 to 60 yards done at half speed, and the speed and distance should be gradually increased over time.

3. To further help avoid injury, you should do your anaerobic training on days when you are rested. One or two days of anaerobic training per week should be sufficient for most people.

Table 7.1 summarizes the anaerobic training principles using FITT.

Table 7.1
Principles of the Anaerobic Training Plan

F—*Frequency:* Perform the anaerobic training program no more than 1 or 2 days per week.

I—*Intensity*: Initially run at a faster than normal pace. Over time, increase intensity to 90% of your maximal heart rate.

T—*Time:* Alternate sprints of 20 to 60 seconds with rest periods twice as long as the exercise time. The number of repetitions will vary depending on the length of the run.

T—*Type of activity*: Any sprint activity (running, swimming, cycling, stair climbing, bounding) could be used, but running is recommended.

Suggested Reading

Chu, D.A. (1992). *Jumping Into Plyometrics.* Champaign, IL: Leisure Press.

PART III

Lifestyle Components of Fitness

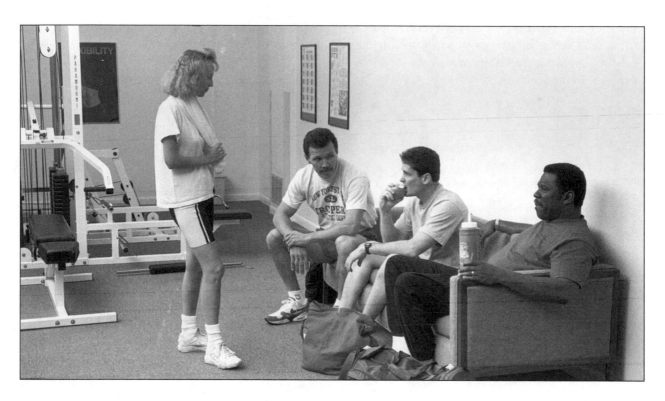

Now you know about the components of physical fitness, and how to develop a program to train each for improved performance and health. But as you learned in chapter 1, there is more to being totally fit than just exercising. This part of the book concentrates on what are commonly called the lifestyle components of fitness.

The lifestyle areas covered in Part III are diet and nutrition, weight management, stress management, smoking cessation, and prevention of substance abuse. Some of you may not have any problems in these areas, and will only need to refer to this section for general information. More likely, however, you may want help in one or more of these areas. Depending on the severity of your problem, you may need professional help beyond the scope of this book.

The purpose of Part III is to give you some general information about the lifestyle components of fitness, help you to understand why law enforcement officers may have problems in some of these areas, and give you some information about where to go for additional help if necessary. It is not intended to be a comprehensive treatment of these complicated subjects. The lifestyle components of fitness will be the subjects of the *FitForce* Fitness Kits. If your agency is a subscriber to the

FitForce Fitness Kits, you can get more detailed information through the kits.

In chapter 8 you will learn about diet and nutrition. Because this subject is a bit more objective than the other lifestyle components, it is more detailed than the other chapters in Part III. Chapter 8 will give you some ideas about what to eat for improved physical performance and health. It will also provide some guidelines for healthier eating.

Directly relating to diet and nutrition and exercise, chapter 9 will discuss weight management. You will learn why it is important to maintain a correct percentage of lean body mass, again for both improved physical performance and health.

According to the American Institute of Stress, being a police officer is the second most stressful job in the nation after that of an inner-city high school teacher. Chapter 10 will discuss some of the stressors contributing to that status, and give you some ideas about where to go for more help.

Law enforcement officers, like everyone else, sometimes react to stress by smoking and abusing substances. Chapter 11 will emphasize the health hazards associated with smoking and present sources of additional help. Chapter 12 in Part III takes a look at substance abuse. In addition to the typical areas of concern—alcohol and drugs—it deals with the problems associated with anabolic steroid usage.

CHAPTER 8

Diet and Nutrition

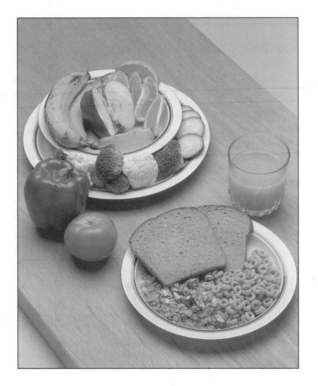

In this chapter you will learn the classes of nutrients and some basic guidelines for healthy eating. You will see how healthy, balanced eating favorably affects your performance and health. Don't worry—you're not going to have to trade all the fun things to eat for seaweed and alfalfa sprouts. Rather, you'll learn to apply balance and moderation and to develop an awareness of what each type of food you encounter can do for you or to you.

Law enforcement officers, with their irregular schedules, find it difficult to maintain healthy eating styles. You are often forced to eat on the run, and as a result fast-food establishments and hot-dog stands meet your needs. Even when you're educated in proper nutritional principles, it can be difficult to eat correctly. So while the information presented in this chapter will give you the nutritional education you need, a more important key to success is changing existing behaviors.

What Is Nutrition?

Diet refers to what is eaten, and nutrition to the value of what is eaten. Specifically, you should be concerned with the impact that food has on body functioning, disease, and weight control.

When you finish this chapter, you will be able to:

✪ Understand how nutrition fits into your overall fitness effort.

✪ Make correct eating choices to enhance both performance and health.

✪ Educate your family about healthy eating.

Classes of Nutrients

There are six classes of nutrients that encompass everything that you eat or drink:

- Carbohydrates
- Minerals
- Vitamins
- Proteins
- Fats
- Water

Each class plays a role in the functioning of your body, and is important to your survival.

Table 8.1 Sources of Carbohydrates		
Grains	**Grain products**	**Secondary sources**
Wheat	Flour	Starches
Rice	Pasta	Potatoes
Corn	Breads	Dry peas
Oats	Breakfast cereals	Vegetables
		Dry beans
		Sugars
		Fruits and juices

Table 8.2 Sources of Fat		
Butter	Cream	Fatty meats
Margarine	Cheeses	Whole milk
Shortening	Nuts	Chocolate
Cooking oils	Bacon	Baked goods
Salad oils	Eggs	Snacks
Mayonnaise		Pastries

Carbohydrates

Carbohydrates are starches, sugars, and fiber. They are the body's primary source of energy; if they aren't available the body uses fats and then protein for energy. Eating sufficient carbohydrates spares proteins so that they can be used for other functions such as building muscles. Carbohydrates also help the body to use fats more efficiently. In addition, the bulk we get from fiber is important for normal health of the intestinal tract, appears to be a factor in reducing the incidence of colon and other cancers, and can help lower the incidence of diabetes. Table 8.1 shows some carbohydrate sources.

A diet high in carbohydrates not only provides energy but also helps you cut down on the amount of fat you eat. (You'll learn more about the health risks of fat later.) The recommended percentage of carbohydrates in the diet is 60% of the total daily intake (see Figure 8.1). The healthiest way to achieve that goal is to increase the amount of carbohydrate-rich foods like whole grain breads, cereals, pasta, fruits, vegetables, and beans in the diet. At the same time, cut back on soft drinks, sweets, and desserts, which have less nutritional value, have no fiber, and cause tooth decay.

Fats

Fats are the most concentrated source of calories of all the nutrients. They have more than twice the amount of energy per unit of weight than either proteins or carbohydrates. But they are not as easy for the body to use for energy as carbohydrates. Fats transport certain vitamins through the body, help build cells, provide insulation, and form a protective cushion around vital organs. Some common sources of fat are listed in Table 8.2.

Cholesterol is a naturally occurring substance in the body that is necessary for certain bodily functions. But too much can be hazardous to your heart. Two lipoproteins (proteins that carry cholesterol through the bloodstream) play a major role in determining whether cholesterol will be harmful to your heart.

The first kind is low-density lipoprotein (LDL), which is bad for your body because it deposits cholesterol on the walls of blood vessels, blocking blood flow (see Figure 8.2). The amount of LDL in your bloodstream is affected by the amount of cholesterol in your diet and is increased by smoking.

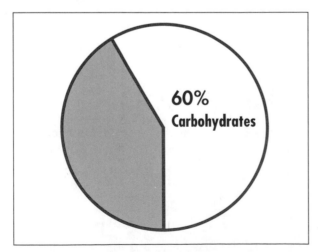

Figure 8.1 *Carbohydrates should comprise 60% of your total daily intake.*

The second kind is high-density lipoprotein (HDL), which is good for your body. It is smaller and denser than LDL. This lipoprotein carries cholesterol to the liver, where it is removed from the bloodstream. It also coats the walls of blood vessels to prevent cholesterol deposits from sticking. The amount of HDL in your bloodstream is not as much affected by dietary cholesterol as the amount of LDL is, but exercise and weight loss can increase HDL levels.

The body makes all the cholesterol that it needs. Because all animal products contain some cholesterol, perhaps more than your body can use, it is important to limit the amount of animal products you eat. This includes the obvious (meat) and the not so obvious (egg yolks). Try to limit your intake to less than 300 mg of cholesterol per day. To put this in perspective, one egg has about 213 mg of cholesterol.

There are two types of fats, saturated and unsaturated. Saturated fats are fats that are solid at room temperature. They are found in foods such as meat, dairy products, eggs, and coconut and palm oils. Avoid these when possible, as they raise your cholesterol level.

Unsaturated fats include monounsaturated and polyunsaturated fats. They are liquid at room temperature. Unsaturated fats help lower cholesterol. Monounsaturated fats are found in olive, canola, and peanut oils. Polyunsaturated fats are in vegetable and fish oils.

In foods that contain both types of fat, such as margarine, choose products that have a ratio of at least three-to-one unsaturated fats to saturated fats. This information is generally available from product labels.

Try to keep the amount of fat in your diet under 30% of your total daily intake (see Figure 8.3). Of those calories, less than one third should be from saturated fat. The best way to do this is to replace red and organ meats with poultry and fish. If you do eat red meats, choose the leaner cuts. Cut down on eggs, oils, and saturated fats. Broil, bake, and boil foods instead of frying them.

To find out what types of fat are in your foods, become a label reader. A lot of informa-tion on food packaging may seem complicated but you can find out almost anything you need from just about any label. For example, most margarines will list total fat content as well as the ratio of saturated and unsaturated fats.

Proteins

These are made up of amino acids, which are the body's building blocks. The body can manufacture about half of the ones it needs; the others must come from food sources. Protein is essential throughout life to build, maintain, and repair tissue. It also makes hemoglobin, which carries oxygen in the blood, and it forms antibodies to fight infection. In an emergency, when carbohydrates and fats are not present,

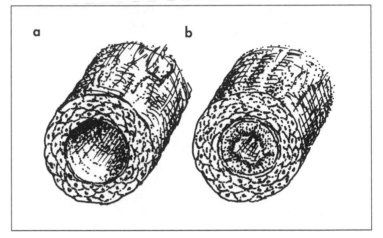

Figure 8.2 *(a) Healthy and (b) unhealthy, clogged arteries.*

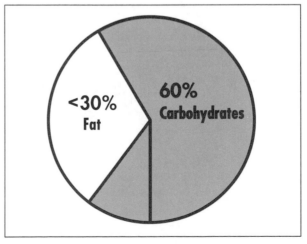

Figure 8.3 *Fat should comprise less than 30% of your daily diet.*

Table 8.3 Sources of Protein	
Foods of animal origin	**Legumes**
Meat	Soybeans
Fish	Chickpeas
Poultry	Lentils
Eggs	Beans
Milk	

the body will use protein for energy. Table 8.3 lists some common protein sources.

The body needs a certain amount of protein every day, but that amount should not exceed 12% of our total daily intake of food (see Figure 8.4). The healthiest way to get sufficient protein is to substitute low-fat foods such as fish, poultry, and low-fat dairy products for red meat and whole-milk products.

Vitamins

While the body only needs very small amounts of vitamins, they are essential for normal functioning. They assist in the release of energy from foods, promote the growth of tissue, and ensure proper functioning of the nerves and muscles. Table 8.4 provides information about vitamins.

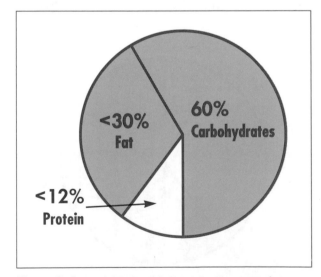

Figure 8.4 *Protein should comprise no more than 12% of your daily intake.*

It's not difficult to get all the vitamins you need in the correct quantities every day by eating balanced meals. If you are in doubt, it's OK to take a daily vitamin supplement. Before buying an expensive name brand, compare its label with that of the generic brands. Generally you'll find that they both give you the same amounts of the recommended daily allowance (RDA). Any brand that gives you 100% of the RDA of the vitamins mentioned in Table 8.4 will probably meet your needs.

Minerals

These are chemical elements the body needs in small quantities. They provide strength and rigidity to certain body tissues and play a part in muscle and nerve function. Table 8.5 gives examples of minerals you need and their sources.

As is true of vitamins, eating a balanced diet will give you your required daily dose of minerals. Again, a daily supplement won't hurt you, and is a good idea for anyone with an iron or calcium deficiency.

Water

Next to oxygen, water is the most important contributor to life. The body is comprised of anywhere from one half to two thirds water. It is the mechanism for the transport of nutrients and the removal of waste products. Water regulates body temperature, aids in digestion, and sustains the health of the cells.

We obviously fulfill some of our need for water with what we drink. We also get it from the foods we eat, especially vegetables, fruits, and meats. Water is also a by-product of energy production within the body.

The thirst mechanism is imperfect, so when you are no longer thirsty you may still not have replaced all the water you have lost. Drink six to eight 8-ounce glasses a day (see Figure 8.5). A word of caution: while all fluids contain water, some are diuretics that cause you to excrete water when you drink them. Alcohol, coffee, tea, and caffeinated soft drinks fall into this category.

Table 8.4 Vitamins		
Vitamin	**Functions**	**Sources**
Vitamin A	Contributes to the visual process and to the formation and maintenance of skin and mucous membranes.	Carrots, sweet potatoes, liver, butter, margarine
Vitamin B	There are eight B vitamins. The three most important are thiamin, riboflavin, and niacin. They assist in the production, metabolism, and utilization of energy.	Whole grains, nuts, milk, yogurt, fish, poultry, cheese, lean pork
Vitamin C	Helps hold cells together and strengthens cell walls. Also has a role in healing wounds and contributes to the maintenance of healthy bones and teeth.	Citrus fruits and juices, broccoli, strawberries, tomatoes, peppers, cauliflower, brussels sprouts, cabbage, potatoes, dark green vegetables, watermelon
Vitamin D	Aids in growth and formation of bones and teeth. Promotes calcium absorption. Vitamin D is also produced by the action of direct sunlight on the skin.	Fortified milk, liver, tuna, eggs
Vitamin E	Protects red blood cells and aids in the metabolism of free fatty acids.	Grains, green leafy vegetables, polyunsaturated fats, vegetable oils
Vitamin K	Assists in blood clotting.	Liver, wheat bran, peas, soybean oil, potatoes

Table 8.5 Important Minerals and Their Sources		
Mineral	**Functions**	**Sources**
Calcium	Gives hardness to teeth and bones. Also involved in nerve and muscle function and the coagulation of blood.	Milk and other dairy products, sardines, dark green vegetables, nuts
Chloride	Assists in cell functioning.	Salt, seafood, milk
Iodine	Prevents goiter.	Iodized salt and seafood
Iron	Combines with protein to form hemoglobin. Helps cells obtain energy from food.	Red meat, liver, shellfish, leafy vegetables, beans, dried fruit
Magnesium	Important for nerve function, bone growth, and muscle contraction.	Whole grains, fruit, leafy vegetables
Phosphorous	Important for formation of bones and teeth, and assists in the transfer of energy.	Meats, poultry, seafood, eggs, milk, beans
Potassium	Important for heart regulation and assists in cell functioning.	Fruits
Sodium	Helps regulate blood pressure.	Salt, seafood, meats

Basic Nutritional Goals

It is virtually impossible to pick up a magazine or newspaper these days without seeing an article about diet and nutrition. Unfortunately, much of the information appears to conflict. This is due in part to the fact that some articles are based on one person's opinion or on research studies with very small sample sizes, and, perhaps most importantly, that everybody's nutritional needs are different. With that in mind, we are not going to overload you with theory, but present some basic nutritional guidelines.

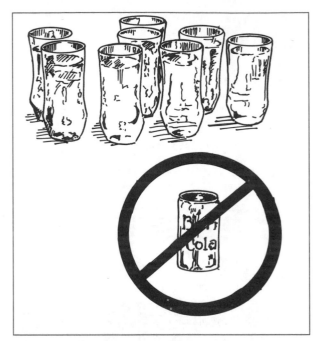

Figure 8.5 *You should drink at least six to eight 8-ounce glasses of water a day.*

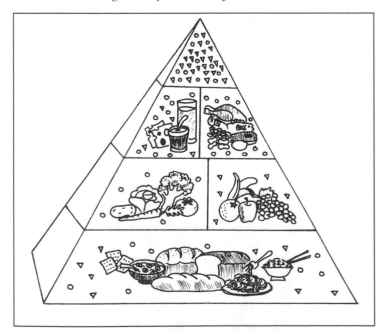

Figure 8.6 *The food pyramid.*

Note. Data from the U.S. Department of Agriculture/U.S. Department of Health and Human Services.

1. Eat three balanced meals a day. Don't skip meals, and make sure that you have the recommended number of servings from each food group as shown in the food pyramid in Figure 8.6. Some people find that eating smaller amounts of food more than three times a day helps them lose weight while curbing appetite.

2. Reduce the amount of all fat, but especially saturated fat in your diet.

3. Lower the cholesterol in your diet. Have your cholesterol measured and periodically rechecked. You want to keep it under 200 mg/dl.

4. Be aware of the amount of sodium in your diet. For some people excessive sodium can raise blood pressure and have other negative impacts on health. Table salt isn't the only culprit here. Be aware of "hidden" sources of sodium, such as catsup, pickles, and processed foods. Read the nutrition labels on the products you buy.

5. Increase the amount of fiber. Eat more fresh fruits, vegetables, bran muffins, and cereals. A word of caution: don't drastically increase the amount of fiber in your diet by eating a day's worth in one sitting or a week's worth in 1 day. This may result in bloating, gas, cramps, or diarrhea.

6. If you are trying to lose weight without much success, keep a very detailed log of exactly what you eat during a week. Using the headings shown in Figure 8.7 will give the type of information you need to analyze your eating habits. You may be surprised how much a little here and a little there can add up to. Also note in your log where and when you eat. You may find that there are certain situations which you need to avoid to help you meet your goal. For example, if eating in front of the television distracts you to the point where you've eaten an entire bag of chips before you realize it, limit your eating to the kitchen.

7. Learn to eat in moderation. You don't have to give up your favorite foods completely,

Date	Time	Food eaten	Amount	Where	Other activity while eating?
6/21	8 p.m.	Potato chips	1 8-oz bag	Den	Watching ball game

Figure 8.7 *Sample headings for eating log.*

even if they aren't the best ones for you nutritionally. Just eat smaller quantities. For example, don't eat the whole bag of a snack food, but rather put a small amount in a bowl and limit yourself to that amount.

8. Eat slowly. Chew your food thoroughly before swallowing, and wait a few minutes before going for that second helping. Most times you'll realize that you aren't as hungry as you may have thought.

9. Learn to make trade-offs. Try eating frozen yogurt instead of ice cream. Get in the habit of eating a piece of fresh fruit instead of chips for a snack. And if you just have to have something crunchy and salty from time to time, pretzels are much lower in fat than are chips.

10. Learn to read labels. Most will give the amounts of each nutrient in a serving, but be careful to identify what the serving size is. Also understand that the ingredients are listed in order of amount, at least through the first five ingredients.

11. If you consume alcohol and caffeine, do so in moderate amounts.

Eating better works for your body like putting higher octane fuel in your car—all other things being equal, it runs better. You'll find that you have more energy, both on and off the job. If you choose to lose weight and achieve it, you will probably see other positive changes. Your movements will become more efficient, so you'll get in and out of your car more easily and climb stairs with less effort. And you will lower your susceptibility to injury, especially to your lower back.

The evidence is overwhelming that following the guidelines put forth earlier have a direct and positive impact on health. A good diet can help reduce our chances of developing diabetes and certain cancers, help us ward off illness, and avoid obesity, which has been very definitely linked to numerous medical problems.

Suggested Readings

Clark, N. (1990). *Nancy Clark's sports nutrition guidebook*. Champaign IL: Leisure Press.

Edwards, T.L. (1988). *Weight loss to super wellness*. Champaign, IL: Human Kinetics.

LeBow, M. (1988). *The thin plan*. Champaign, IL: Human Kinetics.

Thompson, R.A. & Sherman, R.T. (1993) *Helping athletes with eating disorders*. Champaign, IL: Human Kinetics.

Tribole, E. (1992). *Eating on the run*. Champaign, IL: Leisure Press.

CHAPTER 9

Weight Management

Officer Hernandez was told by his doctor that he is 60 pounds overweight. While the number surprised him, he certainly wasn't surprised to find that he was overweight. Virtually every movement, from getting out of bed in the morning to climbing stairs, leaves him huffing and puffing. He even has trouble getting in and out of his patrol car. The few half-hearted attempts he has made to get in shape have ended quickly, in part because strenuous exercise is just too difficult. He has tried a few fad diets, but none of them lasted very long. Is there any hope for Officer Hernandez?

Officer Roberts, on the other hand, wants to gain some strength. She may also want to gain a few pounds of body weight. She wants any weight gain to be muscle, not fat. Can she make that happen?

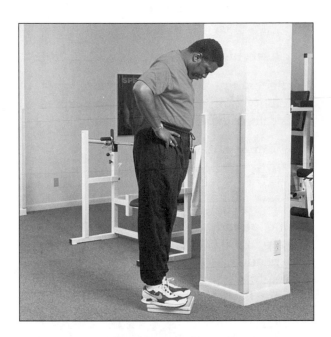

The answer to both of those questions is "yes." In earlier chapters you learned that body composition and body weight are functions of both exercise and diet. This chapter will give you more specific information about weight management.

What Is Weight Management?

A simple way of viewing weight management is to look at the body as an input/output energy system. Weight management is how you balance that energy:

- If the energy in the food eaten equals the energy spent in activity, body weight remains the same.

- If energy put in exceeds the energy put out, body weight increases.

When you finish this chapter, you will be able to:

- ✪ Explain why weight management is an important concept for law enforcement officers.

- ✪ Understand how diet and exercise impact weight management.

- ✪ Apply the principles of energy balance to your weight management program.

- ✪ Determine your goal weight.

- ✪ Know where to go for additional help if weight management is a problem.

- If energy put in is less than the energy put out, body weight decreases.

Here is a brief description of some key concepts relating to energy balance.

- The unit of energy is the calorie (kilocalorie). A kilocalorie is technically one thousand calories, but it is commonly referred to as a calorie.

- Food energy value can be determined and expressed as calorie deposits. For example:

  - 1 serving of oatmeal = 108 calories

  - 1 egg = 79 calories

  - 1 serving of french fries = 220 calories

- The energy demand or energy cost of activity can be determined and expressed as calorie expenditure. For example:

  - Sitting = 105 calories/hour

  - Walking = 345 calories/hour

  - Running = 700 calories/hour

- One pound of fat = 3,500 calories. For every 3,500 calories taken in more than are expended, you will put on 1 pound of weight. For every 3,500 calories expended more than are taken in, you will lose 1 pound of weight.

- Body weight itself is not the most important measurement regarding weight management. Body composition, the ratio of fat to total weight, is more important.

- Body composition is most often expressed as the percentage of fat in the body. For example, a 200-pound person whose percent body fat is estimated at 25% has approximately 50 pounds of fat.

- There are several methods of estimating body fat. They include skinfold measurements, circumference measurements, underwater weighing, electrical impedance, and body mass indexing.

- Guidelines for acceptable body fat vary, but generally match those shown in Table 9.1.

Table 9.1 Body Fat Guidelines		
Category	Men	Women
Ideal	14-17%	21-24%
Overfat	18-19%	25-29%
Borderline obese	20-25%	30-35%
Obesity	>25%	>35%

Why Is Weight Management Important?

Law enforcement officers should be concerned about body fat for its effect on the following:

- Physical performance

- Health

- Appearance

Studies have shown that up to one third of the variance in cardiovascular and muscular endurance is accounted for by the amount of body fat. Thus, maintaining an acceptable level of body fat positively affects physical performance. Other evidence indicates that above a certain level, body fat increases the chance for injury and is linked to other health risks, such as heart disease, high cholesterol, diabetes, cancer, and hypertension.

The appearance issue is more subjective. Does the public have the same confidence in an overweight officer as it does in one who looks fit? Does a perpetrator think that he can "take" an overweight officer? While probably not as important a concern as performance or health, appearance is still an issue.

Principles of Losing Weight

What about Officer Hernandez's problem? As you know, both exercise and diet have an impact on weight loss. The evidence is overwhelming that the most effective weight loss programs involve a combination of both.

Dieting alone doesn't work. When the body is suddenly deprived of the amount of food it is used to getting, it reacts as if it were

Table 9.2			
Caloric Expenditures for Selected Activities			
Activity	Calories/minute	Activity	Calories/minute
Sitting	1.5	Golfing	3.7-5.0
Driving a car	2.8	Rowing	5.0-15.0
House painting	3.5	Cycling (5-15 mph)	5.0-12.0
Raking	4.7	Bowling (while active)	7.0
Weeding	5.6	Handball	10.0
Walking down stairs	7.1	Swimming (leisurely)	6.0
Digging	8.6	Walking (3.5 mph)	5.6-7.0
Walking up stairs	10.0-18.0	Running (5 mph)	10.0

in a starvation situation. It slows down its functions and attempts to conserve energy. Dieters typically lose lean muscle mass as well as fat, so the overall body composition remains the same. Also, dieters tend to go back to their previous eating habits after they lose weight. They quickly gain it back, typically as fat.

Changing your eating habits and increasing your activity are the keys to losing weight and keeping it off. The extra calories burned during exercise, coupled with a reduction of the calories consumed, combine to take off pounds sensibly and steadily. Any activity burns calories and can contribute to weight loss. Walking to the store instead of driving, using the stairs instead of the elevator, and raking leaves are examples of everyday activities you can incorporate into your weight reduction plan.

Officer Hernandez's previous attempts to exercise may have failed because he thought that he needed to do too much. It's ironic that overweight people who need to exercise the most don't do it, at least in part, because they are so poorly conditioned. But Tony now knows that it's OK to start by walking. Once he loses a little weight, it will be possible for him to start jogging, but he doesn't need to run in order to burn calories. Walking, combined with the changes he plans in his eating habits, will be enough to get him started losing weight. To see how much effect small changes can have, take a look at the 500

Plan in Figure 9.1. As a guide for estimating the caloric expenditure of different activities, refer to Table 9.2.

Developing a Weight Management Plan

To control weight and fat gain, follow these steps:

1. Review body composition and body weight. If your agency has a fitness assessment which includes body composition, you will already know both your weight and your percent body fat. If not, look for a health club or health management organization that provides body composition estimation as a service.

One pound of fat contains 3,500 calories. If you divide this by 7, the number of days in the week, you get 500 calories a day. This is the amount that has to be decreased to lose a pound a week or increased to gain a pound a week.

If your weight is above what you want it to be, you should attempt to reduce calories by at least 500 calories a day through exercising and consuming fewer calories. To lose 2 pounds a week, a reduction of 1,000 calories a day is necessary.

If your weight is below what you want it to be, you should eat an additional 500 calories a day to gain a pound a week; 1,000 to gain 2 pounds a week.

For safe and effective weight loss, do not try to lose more than 2 pounds a week.

Figure 9.1 *The 500 Plan.*

An estimate of body composition that you can do yourself is called body mass index (BMI). Figure 9.2 shows how to compute BMI using Officer Hernandez as an example.

2. Establish weight management goals. Calculate your goals for body fat and body weight as part of your goal-setting process (chapter 13). Earlier in this chapter you learned the ideal body fat ranges. Use the following formula to determine your body weight goal:

> **Multiply your body weight times your percent body fat. Fat weight = body weight x % fat (expressed as a decimal).**
>
> **Lean Body Weight (LBW) = weight - fat weight**
>
> **Desired weight = LBW divided by (1 - desired % fat, expressed as a decimal)**
>
> **Desired weight loss = present body weight - desired body weight**

Figure 9.3 shows how Officer Hernandez established his weight management goal.

3. Identify activities for a weight management plan. Many different strategies can be used to develop a weight/fat management plan. It is best to burn or reduce calories by either exercise alone or exercise and diet change. Exercise is more likely to lead to successful weight management because it builds muscles, which require more calories to maintain than fat, and it makes muscles better able to burn fat. It helps maximize the loss of fat and minimize the loss of lean tissue.

4. Implement the weight management program. Planning won't take off a single pound. At some point, you must take action. Easier said than done, but there is only one person who can make it happen—you. Until you gain a feeling for how much you eat, you might want to record your intake and count the calories. There are books available which give the calorie counts for most foods, including fast foods.

There are also many low- or no-fat and low-calorie choices for almost every food product available now. Substitute them as often as possible. Refer to the basic nutritional goals in chapter 8 for other tips on healthy eating.

Tips for Changing Eating Behaviors

Changing behavior is difficult. Your lifestyle consists typically of habits that have been developed over time and have become automatic responses. These following tips may help you with this challenge.

- Monitor yourself. Using a log (similar to the one shown in Figure 8.7) will help you realize how much you eat, what situations trigger overeating, and what substitutions you can make.

- Delay, substitute, or avoid. For example, slow the pace of your eating, go for a walk instead of eating, and spend your break time away from sources of food. After you've eaten, it takes about 20 minutes for the brain to realize you are satisfied.

Officer Hernandez is 70 inches tall and weighs 230 pounds.

1. Convert height and weight to meters (m) and kilograms (kg)

> Height in m = height in inches multiplied by .0254
>
> Weight in kg = weight in pounds divided by 2.2
>
> 70 inches x .0254 = 1.78 m
>
> 230 pounds divided by 2.2 = 105 kg

2. Determine Body Mass Index (BMI)

> BMI = weight (kg) divided by height (m) squared
>
> BMI = 105 divided by (1.78 x 1.78)
>
> BMI = 33.1 kg/m^2

For men, desirable BMI is 22-24 kg/m^2.

For women, desirable BMI is 21-23 kg/m^2.

The risk of cardiovascular disease increases sharply at a BMI of 27.8 kg/m^2 for men and 27.3 kg/m^2 for women.

Figure 9.2 *Computation of body mass index.*

- Reward yourself for changing your behavior. Buy yourself a gift, do something for yourself out of your normal routine, and think positively.

- Ask your family and friends for support. Let them know that you would appreciate their encouragement and that it would help a lot if they didn't put temptations in your path.

- Consider enrolling in a weight management class or program. This would be another source of social support as well as providing helpful information.

Officer Hernandez weighs 230 pounds, with 33% body fat. His intermediate goal is 25%.

1. Multiply body weight times percent body fat

   Fat weight = body weight x % fat (expressed as a decimal)

   Fat weight = 230 x .33

   Fat weight = 76

2. Lean Body Weight (LBW) = weight - fat weight

   LBW = 230 - 76

   LBW = 154

3. Desired weight = LBW divided by (1 - desired % fat, expressed as a decimal)

   Desired weight = 154 divided by (1 - .25)

   Desired weight = 154 divided by .75

   Desired weight = 205

4. Desired weight loss = present body weight - desired body weight

   Desired weight loss = 233 - 205

   Desired weight loss = 28 pounds

Figure 9.3 *Officer Hernandez's weight management goal.*

While not everyone has a weight problem, almost everyone deals with the issue of weight control at one time or another. As with the other components of a total fitness program, it interfaces with each of the others. You have already seen the connections with exercise and diet and nutrition. In the next chapter you will learn about stress. For many people, weight management is one of the most stressful parts of their lives. As you will see, the positive effects of maintaining a healthy body weight can go beyond improved performance and physical health, and it may positively influence your mental health as well.

Suggested Readings

Since the best way to lose unwanted weight is a combination of aerobic exercise and sensible eating, all of the additional readings in chapters 4 and 8 are applicable. The following titles are also recommended.

Cotterman, S.K. (1985). *Y's way to weight management.* Champaign, IL: Human Kinetics.

LeBow, M.D. (1988). *The thin plan.* Champaign, IL: Human Kinetics.

Malina, R.M., & Bouchard, C. (1991). *Growth, maturation, and physical activity.* Champaign, IL: Human Kinetics.

Sharkey, B.J. (1990). *Physiology of fitness.* Champaign, IL: Human Kinetics.

Shephard, R.J. (1994). *Aerobic fitness and health.* Champaign, IL: Human Kinetics.

Storlie, J., & Jordan, H. (1984). *Behavioral management of obesity.* Champaign, IL: Human Kinetics.

Storlie, J., & Jordan, H. (1984). *Evaluation and treatment of obesity.* Champaign, IL: Human Kinetics.

Storlie, J., & Jordan, H. (1984). *Nutrition and exercise in obesity management.* Champaign, IL: Human Kinetics.

CHAPTER 10

Stress Management

H ave you ever

- been driving to work when the traffic came to a standstill because of an accident?

- felt that the demands of your job were building to the point where you just couldn't take it anymore?

- had a domestic disturbance escalate to the point where you were threatened with weapons?

You've probably experienced more than one of these examples, and could list lots of similar events. In addition to recognizing that there will always be some amount of stress in

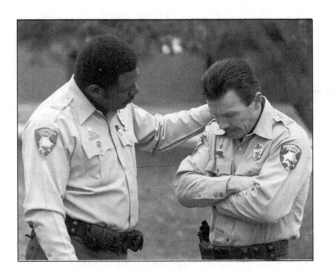

your life, it is also important to recognize the signs that the stressors in your life are causing negative reactions. Chances are that when you were experiencing these events, you also noted some of the following physical changes:

- Increased heart rate
- Nervousness
- Faster breathing
- Sweaty palms
- Headaches

- Irritability
- Indigestion
- Trouble sleeping
- Weight fluctuation

What Is Stress?

What you were experiencing in these and similar situations was stress. Stress can occur when outside conditions cause physical and mental reactions. You perceive that the requirements of the conditions are beyond your capacity to deal with them. Your reaction

When you finish this chapter you will be able to:

- ✪ Explain why law enforcement work presents special stressors.

- ✪ Understand that negative responses to stress have an unfavorable impact on both performance and health.

- ✪ Recognize that you have both avoidable and unavoidable stressors in your life and learn ways to cope with them.

- ✪ Understand that exercise is an effective stress management tool.

- ✪ Know where to seek additional help with stress-related problems.

to the situation depends upon how important the outcome is to you. If it is important, you experience stress. How you handle your reactions determines to what extent the stress affects your performance and health.

Dealing With Stress

People deal with stress in various ways. For instance, you can allow stress to have a negative effect. Consider this example:

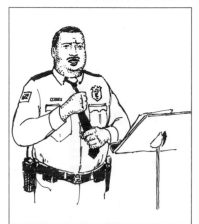

Officer Hernandez had a presentation to make to the chief. Of course he wanted to do well, but he was so nervous about how he would come across that he didn't sleep well for several nights before the meeting. Resorting to his familiar "coping strategies," he temporarily relieved his tension by drinking after work. This caused trouble at home, which in turn caused him to accuse his wife of not understanding the pressure he was under. By the time he gave his presentation, he was convinced that he would do poorly, and he flubbed several parts of the briefing. In this case, Officer Hernandez allowed the stress to be destructive.

You can also take control of your stress and use it to improve your performance. When Officer Roberts had to make a presentation to her boss, she saw it as an opportunity to shine. She had been looking for a chance to show the chief that she had what it took for promotion to the next grade. Thus energized,

Monique organized her presentation early, rehearsed until she was comfortable with her delivery, and was excited about the opportunity. As a result, she went into the meeting confident and rested, and her presentation went very smoothly. In this case, Officer Roberts used the stress as a positive to psyche herself up and perform better than she might have without pressure.

Everyone experiences stress; it's a part of living. The key is learning to manage it. By practicing ways to deal with stress positively, you can:

- Improve your performance by eliminating distracting worries

- Prevent a series of minor stressors from building up your stress to a high level

- Become better able to handle daily stressors

Relationship Between Stress and Health

Several studies have suggested that law enforcement is significantly more stressful than other occupations, including fire fighting. There are also indications that health problems such as elevated blood pressure, cardiovascular disease, lower-back pain, and gastrointestinal disorders are stress-related physical health problems common to law enforcement officers. Data show that law enforcement officers have a high incidence of stress-related emotional problems such as suicide, divorce, and alcoholism.

Some of the stressors associated with law enforcement are obvious but unavoidable, such as confrontations with dangerous people

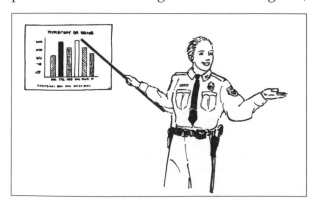

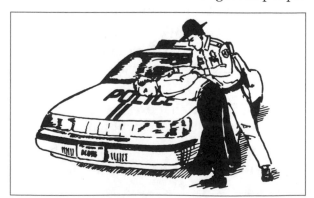

in life-threatening situations, the noise and pollution associated with traffic, and the long hours which keep you away from your family and friends.

There are also less obvious stressors. For example, sometimes your job requires long hours of inactivity and boredom. Inactivity is both a cause and effect of stress. Spending the greater part of every day sitting and waiting for something to happen can contribute to a buildup of stress. Over time, the body's ability to adapt to this type of stress deteriorates, and it becomes difficult to find the energy and enthusiasm to participate in activity outside of work. Therefore, the stress contributes to further inactivity, which in turn causes more stress.

Effects of Exercise on Stress

The best way to break out of this vicious cycle is to exercise. Exercise has been shown to be an effective way to reduce stress. There are two major benefits of an exercise program as an element of stress management. First, by doing something about the problem, you take control, and taking control builds self-esteem. Research has shown that officers with high self-esteem have fewer stress-related problems.

Second, regular exercise helps you maintain the energy necessary to adapt to and handle stress over time. It breaks the vicious cycle of inactivity leading to stress, and vice versa. A long-term exercise program appears to reduce the bad effects of stress. Fit individuals who exercise appear more relaxed and confident, and less anxious. Active individuals report less stress and tension, and one study found that exercise was significantly more effective than tranquilizers for reducing the anxiety-tension state associated with stress.

Avoidable and Unavoidable Stressors

Another way to manage stress is to think about the stressors in your life and plan ways to avoid them or make them less stressful. First, identify the negative stressors, using Figure 10.1. Examine your day-to-day activities closely, and try to uncover even the least obvious. Your strategy will be different for each set of activities.

For example, Officer Johnson's lists started like this:

Avoidable Stressors	Plan
Listening to Officer Jones complain every day at lunch	_____ _____ _____

Unavoidable Stressors	Coping Strategy
30-minute ride to work	_____ _____ _____

You will want to come up with a plan to deal with the avoidable stressors. For example, if every time you get with certain people you have a political argument which raises your blood pressure, try to avoid those people. Or if the inactivity of certain aspects of your job is causing your fitness level to deteriorate to a point where you have entered the vicious circle we talked about before, start a fitness program.

What about the stressors that are unavoidable? For each of these, you want to develop and adapt a coping strategy (see Figure 10.2). That is, you acknowledge that they are inevitable but that you are going to minimize the effect they will have on you. Just recognizing that there will always be stressors in your life is an important first step

Stressor	Plan
_____	_____
_____	_____
_____	_____
_____	_____
_____	_____

Figure 10.1 *Avoidable stressors.*

that can help you to deal with them better. The next step is to develop a message to give yourself about the event, a message which helps to place it into perspective. For example, when you are forced to spend more time away from the family than you like, keep telling yourself about the attention you are going to give them when you do see them again.

Let's go back to our example and see how Officer Johnson decided to deal with his avoidable and unavoidable stressors:

Avoidable Stressors	Plan
Listening to Officer Jones complain every day at lunch	Change my lunch schedule

Unavoidable Stressors	Coping Strategy
30-minute ride to work	Listen to those self-improvement tapes I never find time for at home

Relaxation Techniques

Another technique to help you deal with stress is to learn to relax. A training exercise that you can use is to alternately and systematically tense and relax parts of your body. This exercise has two aims: (a) to help you learn how to relax and (b) to help you learn to recognize when your muscles are becoming tense.

Stressor	Coping Strategy
_____	_____
_____	_____
_____	_____
_____	_____
_____	_____

Figure 10.2 *Unavoidable stressors.*

Lie down in a quiet, semi-dark room. Take a few deep breaths. Starting with one foot, tense it for about 10 seconds. As you relax your foot, feel the tension flowing out of the area. Concentrate on the difference between the feelings of tension and relaxation. Now follow the same sequence with your other foot, again concentrating as the tension ebbs away. Next alternate the legs, then your buttocks, each hand, the arms, your neck, face, and finally the whole body. Lie quietly after the last relaxation and concentrate on what you are feeling.

While some people will immediately feel relaxed to the point of drowsiness from this exercise, others will need a few more sessions to achieve the desired effect. Try this exercise on a regular basis when you feel tension building up in one part of your body. With practice you will be able to recognize the onset of tension and be able to eliminate it before it spreads and tightens up your entire body.

Additional Tips for Reducing Stress

Other thoughts to consider for reducing stress are:

- Share your feelings with someone you trust.

- Take care of your body, as well as your mind. All the negative aspects of stress are amplified if you are unhealthy.

- Get away from the everyday routine whenever possible.

- Don't put unrealistic demands upon yourself. Recognize your limits, and strive to do the best you can with what you've got.

This chapter has given you a brief introduction to a very complicated subject. It is beyond the scope of this book to delve deeper into it. There are many books written on the subject, and the titles of some of them are provided for you. You may feel that you need some additional information or help. Perhaps your agency has a counselor on staff, or maintains a relationship with one who specializes in the treatment of law enforcement stress.

The key to stress management is to control the stressors in your life and not let them control you. Start an exercise program to avoid the vicious circle of inactivity leading to stress which then results in more inactivity. Develop a plan to avoid the unnecessary stressors. Prepare yourself to meet the stressors which are unavoidable. Finally, learn to relax.

Suggested Readings

Coulson, R. (1993). *Police under pressure: Resolving disputes.* Westport, CT: Greenwood.

Drake B.M., Inc. (1993). *Managing stress in turbulent times.* New York: D B M Publishing.

Eliot, R.S. (1994). *A change of heart: Converting your stresses to strengths.* New York: Bantam Books.

Johnson, C.S., & Johnson, R.L. (1993).*Stress & anger management.* Pasco, WA: Life Choices.

Lehrer, P.M., & Woolfolk, R.L. (1993). *Principles & practices of stress management.* (2nd Ed.) New York: Guilford Press.

McQuade, W., & Aikman, A. (1993). *Stress: What it is, what it can do to your health, how to handle it.* New York: NAL/Dutton.

Miskell, V., & Miskell, J.R. (1994). *Overcoming anxiety at work.* Burr Ridge, IL: Irwin Professional Publishing.

O'Hara, V. (1990). *The fitness option: Five weeks to healing stress.* Nevada City, CA: Dawn Publications.

Olesen, E. (1993). *Twelve steps to mastering the winds of change: Peak performers reveal how to stay on top in times of turmoil.* New York: Macmillan.

Toner, P.R. (1993). *Stress management & self-esteem activities.* West Nyack, NY: Center for Applied Research in Education.

Wright, M. (1994). *A handbook of stress for careers.* New York: Cassell.

Youngs, B.B. (1993). *A stress management guide for administrators.* Torrance, CA: Jalmar Press.

CHAPTER 11

Smoking Cessation

Smoking is one of the largest barriers to a smoker's total fitness. Tobacco smoking is linked to heart attacks, stroke, lung and other types of cancer, emphysema, and chronic bronchitis. It also reduces the capacity to exercise because it restricts lung function and cuts down on the amount of oxygen that reaches the muscles and organs.

Tobacco use is one of the most powerful addictions known to man. Despite the overwhelming evidence that it is the number one killer in America today, 45 million Americans still smoke. There is evidence that law enforcement officers smoke at a greater rate than the general population.

The number of smokers includes otherwise intelligent, well-informed persons who either can't or won't quit. Some continue to deny the possibility that smoking is bad for them. If you are a smoker, you may find these statistics enlightening:

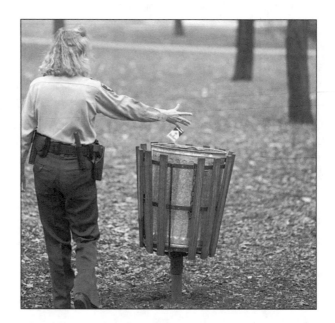

- Each year nearly 400,000 Americans die from diseases related to smoking:

  115,000 from coronary heart disease

  27,000 from stroke

  136,000 from cancer

  60,000 from chronic pulmonary disease

  50,000 from other diseases

- Out of 100 persons who try to quit smoking, 60 go back to smoking before the first year is out.

- Smoking accounts each year for $22 billion in medical costs and another $43 billion in lost production.

- Medicare and Medicaid alone pay out over $4 billion to care for those who are ill from cigarette-related diseases.

When you finish this chapter, you will be able to:

- ✪ Recognize that smoking is detrimental to your performance and health.

- ✪ Understand why smoking is harmful.

- ✪ Recognize that this topic is important to you even if you don't smoke.

- ✪ Explain the benefits of quitting.

- ✪ Know where to go for help if you need it.

- Smoking doubles the risk for heart disease. Coupled with hypertension or high cholesterol, the risk is four times greater. Combined with both, the risk is eight times greater.

- Some 30% of all cancer deaths, and 90% of lung cancer deaths, are due to smoking.

- More than 2 million persons suffer from emphysema, 500,000 so severely that they cannot work or maintain a household.

- Exposure to tobacco smoke poses grave risks to babies, both before and after they are born.

- Smokers run a greater risk of premature death than do nonsmokers (see Figure 11.1).

What's So Bad About Cigarettes?

The harm caused by cigarettes is due to what is in the smoke and to the excessive exposure a smoker has to the smoke. A two-pack-a-day smoker spends from 3 to 4 hours a day with a cigarette in hand, mouth, or ashtray. She or he takes about 400 puffs, and inhales up to 1,000 milligrams of tar.

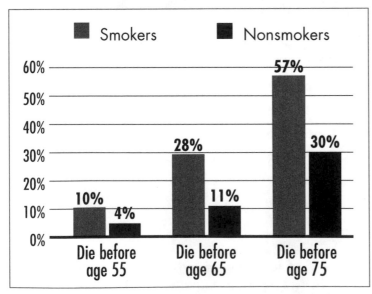

Figure 11.1 *Smokers run a greater risk of premature death than do nonsmokers.*

Note. Data from *Smoking tobacco and health,* Centers for Disease Control (1989), p. 9.

Tar is the oily material left after the smoke has passed through the filter. It consists of over 4,000 chemical substances. Forty-three of these are known to cause or promote cancer, and 401 others are toxic or harmful in other ways. There is no safe level of exposure for many of them.

Hemoglobin is a part of the blood which carries oxygen to the working muscles. One of the gasses in tobacco smoke, carbon monoxide, bonds with hemoglobin to form carboxyhemoglobin. This, in turn, diminishes the blood's ability to carry oxygen. High enough concentrations of carbon monoxide can cause death. Smokers have levels of carboxyhemoglobin from 2 to 15 times higher than nonsmokers.

Nicotine is a highly addictive drug produced by the tobacco plant. In large doses it is extremely poisonous. It can have different effects on the body in different situations. Sometimes it acts as a calming agent, for instance in stressful situations. At other times it may act as a stimulant. This may partly explain smoking patterns, as smokers meet their need for this drug in different ways. For example, the high stress of law enforcement work may make the calming effect of smoking desirable in those stressful situations.

The more a person smokes, the greater the risk of smoking-related diseases. Two-pack-a-day smokers are six times more likely to die of lung cancer than are those who smoke a half a pack a day. In addition to the number of cigarettes smoked, other factors such as the number of puffs and how deeply the smoke is inhaled influence the effects of smoking.

Effects of Second-Hand Smoke

The effects of second-hand smoke are being hotly debated. In the presence of smokers, nonsmokers absorb carbon dioxide, nicotine, and other by-products of smoke, just as smokers do. Heavy exposure may have the same impact as smoking two cigarettes a day would. Besides being annoying to some, it physically affects others. Exposure to second-hand smoke can worsen the symptoms of asthma, chronic bronchitis, and allergies.

To protect the health rights of nonsmokers, smoking has become an organizational policy area. Smoking bans are increasingly acceptable as facility and employment standards. Consequently, smoking cessation is an important area for fitness lifestyle educational programming.

Benefits of Quitting

Those who quit smoking can reap many health benefits:

- Lung cancer risk drops to almost half that of smokers after 10 years and continues to decrease.

- After 1 year of quitting, smokers' excess risk (beyond that of nonsmokers) of heart disease is cut in half. After 15 years, the risk is the same as if they had never smoked.

- In 5 to 15 years, the risk of stroke also returns to the level of those who have never smoked.

- Health status is much better than that of smokers. Those who quit have fewer sick days and health complaints, report better health, and have a lower incidence of bronchitis and pneumonia.

- After 15 years off cigarettes, the risk of death for ex-smokers returns to nearly the level of persons who have never smoked.

- Male smokers who quit between ages 35 to 39 add an average of 5 years to their lives. Female quitters in this age group add 3 years.

    There are also non–health-related benefits:

- Cigarettes are expensive, and due to become more so. Ex-smokers save money.

- With the increasing number of places banning smoking, life is more convenient.

- Food tastes better, as taste buds are no longer desensitized.

- Exercise becomes easier due to the improved performance of the cardiovascular system.

- Your clothes and hair won't smell like smoke. Neither will your breath, and the yellowing of your teeth caused by nicotine will be eliminated.

How Do You Quit?

Quitting is hard. According to a recent Gallup poll, more than 75% of smokers have tried to quit smoking. Their success rates are not positive. They remained smoke-free as follows:

Less than a month	44%
1-3 months	22%
More than 3 months	32%

Presenting a prescription for quitting is beyond the scope of this book. For many, quitting without professional assistance is impossible. Organizations providing professional services are listed in Appendix C.

If you do smoke and think you can quit by yourself, try the following steps.

1. Review your current smoking habits. Assess the level of nicotine dependence, using the Fagerstrom Tolerance Test shown in Figure 11.2. As a general rule, high dependence will require professional assistance to quit.

2. Establish a smoking-cessation goal. This is accomplished through choosing a quitting goal and a date for beginning to work toward that goal. For some individuals, gradual tapering off needs to be the initial goal.

3. Develop a smoking-cessation plan. Many programs are marketed to aid in smoking cessation. SmokEnders, American Heart, and the "patch" are just a few. A recent report in the *Journal of the American Medical Association* says that using nicotine patches can double a smoker's prospects for successfully quitting. Research found that 27% of patients ceased smoking while wearing the patch, compared to 13% using placebos. Other findings about the patch were that 16-hour and 24-hour patches seem to work equally well, and that "weaning" with gradually weaker patches doesn't make quitting more likely.

Your local American Heart Association, American Lung Association, and American Cancer Society can supply many resources, some of which are free.

4. Implement the program. Implementing the smoking-cessation program involves monitoring the daily smoking count (how many cigarettes smoked) and using various behavior control strategies such as contracting, which will be discussed in chapter 14.

The best advice about smoking: If you haven't started, don't. But if you have, it's never too late to gain the benefits available from quitting.

Check off the answer to each question.

Questions	Answers	Point Score
1. How soon after you wake do you smoke your first cigarette?	Within 30 minutes	1 _____
	After 30 minutes	0 _____
2. Do you find it difficult to refrain from smoking in places where it is forbidden?	Yes	1 _____
	No	0 _____
3. Which cigarette would you hate to give up the most?	The first one in the morning	1 _____
	Any other	0 _____
4. How many cigarettes a day do you smoke?	15 or less	0 _____
	16-25	1 _____
	26 or more	2 _____
5. Do you smoke more frequently during the early morning than during the rest of the day?	Yes	1 _____
	No	0 _____
6. Do you smoke if you are so ill that you are in bed most of the day?	Yes	1 _____
	No	0 _____
7. What is the nicotine level of your usual brand of cigarettes?	0.9 mg or less	0 _____
	1.0-1.2 mg	1 _____
	1.3 mg or more	2 _____
8. Do you inhale?	Never	0 _____
	Sometimes	1 _____
	Always	2 _____
	Total	_____

Scoring for the Fagerstrom Tolerance Test

Total your points. A score of 7 or higher indicates high nicotine dependence; a score of 6 or lower indicates low to moderate nicotine dependence.

Figure 11.2 *The Fagerstrom Tolerance Test.*

Suggested Readings

Centers for Disease Control. (1989). *Smoking tobacco & health* (DHHS Publication No. [CDC] 87-8397). Washington, DC: U.S. Government Printing Office.

Jones, K.Z. (1993). *Help someone you love quit smoking*. New York: Putnam.

Krumholz, H. & Phillips, R.H. (1993). *No if's, and's, or butts: A smoker's guide to quitting*. Garden City, NY: Avery Publishing Group.

Voss, T. (1993). *Smoking and common sense: One doctor's view*. Concord, MA: Paul and Company Publishers Consortium.

CHAPTER 12

Substance Abuse Prevention

Officer Hernandez likes to have a few drinks with his buddies after work. He doesn't drink heavily; nevertheless, his wife is not always happy to see him when he gets home.

Officer Roberts's sister Ruth likes to smoke a few joints with her friends. Besides being against the law, it seems to affect her personality. She used to be the most popular girl in her class. Now many of her old friends don't want to have anything to do with her.

Officer Johnson's son Reggie wants to make the varsity football team next year. He's been going to the weight room regularly during the off-season. Some of the guys have made dramatic improvements in their size and strength. They've told Reggie that the improvements come from using anabolic steroids. Reggie feels that he won't be able to compete for a position on the team if he doesn't use them also.

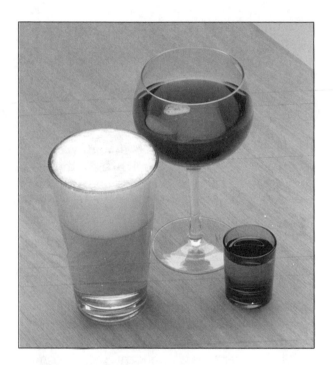

Each of these scenarios is common. They all reflect possibilities for the abuse of substances. In some cases the substances are illegal, like the pot and the steroids, and in others they are legal, like alcohol and prescription drugs. But in either case there is potential for misuse which can destroy careers, families, and the individuals themselves. As an officer, you are concerned with this issue from several different perspectives:

- Your own well-being
- The well-being of your family
- The public you serve
- The law you are sworn to uphold

When you finish this chapter, you will be able to:

- ✪ Understand why substance abuse is harmful to both your performance and health.

- ✪ Recognize some signs and symptoms of different types of substance abuse.

- ✪ Know where to go for help if you need it.

Areas of Concern Regarding Substance Abuse

There are three main areas where substance abuse comes into play: legal, social, and health. You are abundantly familiar with the legal implications. The societal implications are important within the scope of this book from a stress management point of view. Therefore, this section will concentrate on the health and performance effects of the three primary substances most likely to be abused by you and your family: alcohol, drugs (both recreational and prescription), and steroids (technically a drug, but used for a different purpose than we commonly think of when we address the "drug problem").

Alcohol

The abuse of alcohol affects many lives in the United States. As with all drugs, there are legal, social, and health consequences associated with its misuse. While alcohol use itself is legal, every day thousands of Americans break the law by getting behind the wheel of a vehicle with a blood-alcohol content above the legal limit. While few people who do this equate it with a burglary or other crime, it is no less illegal, and the potential consequences are horrible to consider. Fully one half of all the motor vehicle accidents in the U.S. involve alcohol. Every day, innocent men, women, and children are struck down before their time by drunk drivers. The public outrage has grown to the point that laws are becoming stricter. The amount of alcohol in the blood required to declare someone under the influence gets lower with the passage of tougher legislation.

There are other problems associated with the abuse of alcohol. Many families are destroyed because of the destructive use of alcohol by one or more members. By some definitions, use of alcohol in any quantity is a problem if it affects family life. That means if Officer Hernandez's wife gets upset because he has one beer on the way home from work, then alcohol use is a problem for his family.

More familiarly recognized as problem behavior is domestic violence resulting from drinking. How many calls have you answered for this problem? And as you well know, the scenario may involve anything from disturbing the neighbors to spouse abuse.

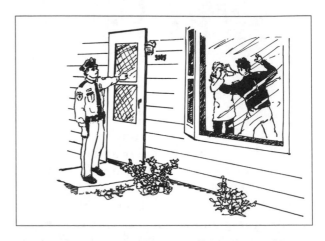

Problems with drinking often carry over to the job and manifest themselves in different ways. Drinkers are more often late for work, and over time usually develop attendance problems. Their performance on the job deteriorates as they deal with drowsiness, headaches, lack of concentration, and other symptoms of hangovers. Their appearance may be affected, and being around them may become offensive to the senses of their fellow employees.

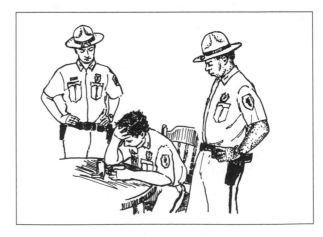

About 7% of American adults can be categorized as alcohol abusers or as alcohol dependent. Alcohol consumption increases with income, and is more prevalent among males than among females. There appears to be a genetic component to alcoholism; that is, offspring of alcoholics are at high risk of becoming alcoholics themselves.

Alcohol is often available in social settings, and there is nothing wrong with being a social drinker. Unfortunately, many people have forgotten how to drink socially. Here are a few tips on drinking socially.

- Never accept a drink unless you want one.

- Know your limit.

- Eat while you drink.

- Sip your drinks, don't gulp them.

- Alternate alcoholic and nonalcoholic beverages.

- Don't drink to relax.

- Don't drink to forget your problems.

- Don't drink and drive.

Finally, there is the health issue. While generally considered to be underreported, alcohol-related illnesses are still responsible for 3% of deaths in America each year. Certain cancers, liver damage, impotency, and other nerve disorders have all been connected with alcohol abuse. It also causes digestive abnormalities which can result in nutritional deficiencies. In addition, alcohol blocks the ability of the blood to carry oxygen to the working muscles by attaching to hemoglobin, the oxygen-carrying element of the blood. This detracts from performance in all activities requiring cardiovascular endurance.

Generally, people with drinking problems need professional help to quit. The all-important first step is recognition of the problem. The tendency is to deny that a problem exists and to claim that you can stop at any time. There are any number of tools to use to make an assessment of whether or not alcohol is a problem in your life. One such tool is the checklist in Figure 12.1.

If you answered "yes" to any of these questions, you may have a problem with alcohol. You should see a counselor for more definitive guidance.

Drugs

We all know that the use of street drugs (or recreational drugs) is against the law. We also have been exposed to enough information that we know the harm street drugs can do to our health. We read in the paper every day about someone dying from an overdose. The statistics relating crime to drug use are staggering. Yet people continue to use and abuse drugs. Why? Because they are so powerfully addictive that the only sure way to stay off of drugs is to never get on them to begin with.

As with alcohol, treatment is best left with a professional. Recognizing a problem with either yourself or someone you care about is again the critical first step. The more difficult step is doing something about it.

While so far we have concentrated on illegal drugs, the abuse of prescription drugs is no less harmful. They can have the same debilitating effects on health, performance, and relationships as do street drugs. In some ways there may be more potential for danger, because often the abusers are otherwise law-

---

Answer "yes" or "no" to the following questions.

_____ Do you ever drink alone?

_____ Do you ever drink when you first get up in the morning?

_____ Do you ever forget things you did while you were drinking?

_____ Have you ever missed work because of drinking?

_____ Do you have a drink to get ready to face certain situations?

_____ Do you push others to drink when they may not want to?

_____ Do you avoid events where alcohol will not be served?

_____ Do you deny how much you drink?

_____ Do you lie about drinking?

_____ Do you drink large amounts and feel no effect the next day?

If you answered "yes" to any of these questions, you may have a problem with alcohol.

Figure 12.1 *Alcohol-abuse checklist.*

abiding people who may never be suspected of having this problem and may not realize it themselves.

We will assume that drug abuse is not a problem for the readers of this book but that it may be for people they care about. Some signs that a person is having a problem with drugs include the following behavioral changes:

- Keeping odd hours
- Otherwise unexplained loss of weight
- Personality change—becoming withdrawn
- Loss of interest in school, work, and other activities
- Deterioration of appearance

There are any number of counseling services available for those with drug abuse problems. The biggest problem is getting the individual to admit that he or she needs help. Having someone who cares makes it much easier to face up to the problem and try to do something about it. While this can be a very trying time for all concerned, the following tips may help you deal with the situation a little bit better:

- Don't try to deal with someone under the influence.
- Don't cover up or make excuses for the person.
- Don't make an issue about seeking treatment.
- Provide a supportive home environment.
- Don't expect overnight changes.

Steroids

The estimates of steroid use among young American males are frightening. Despite the well-publicized destructive results of using steroids for anything other than prescribed medical purposes, many are unable to think of anything other than the short-term gains in strength and size available. Steroid use can result in severe physical, as well as psychological, changes. These include increased cholesterol, triglycerides, and glucose; shrunken testicles; irritability; and "'roid rage." Education is a key. Youngsters seeing the short-term results of steroid usage are going to have a hard time accepting the long-term price to be paid without some good guidance and education. Steroid use increases the risk of liver cancer, hepatitis, hypertension, and diabetes.

Symptoms of steroid use include:

- Mood swings and increased aggressiveness
- Acne
- Voice lowering (in females)
- Increase in facial and body hair
- Above-normal gains in muscle mass

This chapter only scratches the surface of the issues surrounding substance abuse. As noted, many substance abuse problems require professional help. You now have some additional information that hopefully you will never need. Unfortunately, that is probably not realistic. If you do suspect a problem, taking some action is better than sitting back and letting the problem worsen, whether it's yours or someone else's.

Suggested Readings

Bean, R. *Drugs and alcohol: Helping children avoid substance abuse*. Price Stern Sloan.

Brandeis University, Institute for Health Policy Staff. (1993). *Substance abuse: The nation's number one health problem*. Princeton, NJ: The Robert Wood Johnson Foundation.

Freeman, E.M. (Ed.). (1993). *Substance abuse treatment: A family systems perspective*. Newbury Park, CA: Sage Publications, Incorporated.

Heinemann, A.W. (Ed.). (1993). *Substance abuse and physical disability*. New York: The Haworth Press Incorporated.

Korenman, S.G., & Barchas, J.D. (Eds.). (1993). *Biological basis of substance abuse*. NewYork: Oxford University Press.

Lewis, J.A., Dana, R.Q., & Blevins, G.A. (1994). *Substance abuse counseling: An individual approach*. Pacific Grove, CA: Brooks/Cole Publishing Company.

Muisener, P.P. (1994). *Understanding & treating adolescent substance abuse*. Thousand Oaks, CA: Sage Publications.

O'Farrell, T.J. (Ed.). (1993). *Treating alcohol problems: Marital and family interventions*. New York: Guilford Press.

Oryx Press Staff. (Ed.). (1993). *Drugs, alcohol, and other addictions: A directory of treatment centers & preventions programs nationwide* (2nd ed.). Phoenix: Oryx Press.

Shoker, N. (1993). *Substance abuse*. New York: Chelsea House Publishers.

Straussner, S.L. (Ed.). (1992). *Clinical work with substance-abusing clients*. New York: Guilford Press.

Toner, P.R. (1993). *Substance abuse prevention activities*. West Nyade, NY: The Center for Applied Research in Education.

Yesalis, C.E. (Ed.) (1993). *Anabolic steroids in sport and exercise*. Champaign IL: Human Kinetics.

Setting Course and Staying With It

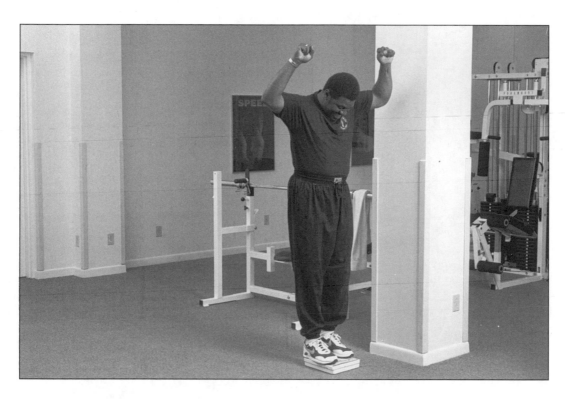

Now you have the information you need to get started on a fitness program to improve health and performance. Part I helped you to determine your current level of physical fitness, and gave you a starting point to build from. Part II gave you all the information you need to design a program to improve your cardiovascular endurance, muscular strength and endurance, flexibility, and anaerobic power. In Part III, you learned some basic information about the lifestyle components of fitness.

Part IV will tie all the previous information together. You were exposed to some elements of goal setting in chapters 4 through 7.

Chapter 13 will present a more formal approach to this key subject. You will learn why it is important to set goals, both for fitness and in other areas of your life. Using examples based on Officers Hernandez, Johnson, and Roberts, you will be able to follow the goal-setting procedure as you learn the principles. There are forms included which will facilitate your own goal-setting process.

Even the most dedicated, experienced exercisers have days when they find it hard to get started. People also fall off of their programs occasionally for reasons beyond their control, such as injuries. The purpose of chapter 14 is to give you some cautions about potential pitfalls and sidetracks in your fitness efforts. It will give you some motivational tools to use at those times when you may need a boost. You will also learn about fitness contracts, and how they may help you adhere to your program.

Goal Setting

In chapter 2, you learned about fitness assessments. In Part II, you learned how to train using the components of physical fitness. Part III gave you some information about the lifestyle components of fitness. Throughout those chapters, you gained some insights into what kind of goals you might consider for your own program. The purpose of this chapter is to give you some more specific information about the process of goal setting. You'll be focusing on fitness goals to define the expectations for maintaining and improving fitness, but goal setting can help you in all areas of your life, not just your fitness program.

Most of us perform better when we have a specific goal to work toward. A goal gives meaning to our actions, helps establish intermediate benchmarks to check progress, and provides motivation. Studies have shown that people have greater adherence to programs when they set goals, and the adherence is even stronger when they write their goals down.

Goal setting should be an ongoing, systematic, and progressive process. As you

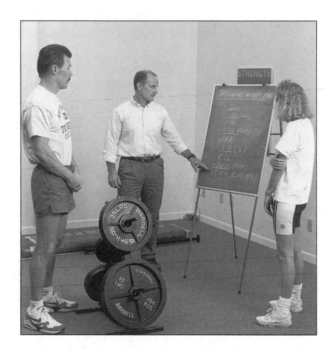

learn more about your abilities, you may want to update your goals to make them more realistic. And as you attain a goal, set a new challenge for yourself. Your expectations should just exceed your reach!

Developing Goals

To develop goals, you must know where you are now, have some idea of where you want to go, consider what it's going to take to get there, and have a way to evaluate your progress. Here are four steps to help you visualize this process.

Step 1: Know where you are now. There are several ways to evaluate your present condition. One would be the assessments you did

When you finish this chapter, you will be able to:

✪ Know why goals are important.

✪ Understand how the goal-setting process works.

✪ Develop your goals.

✪ Know when to change your goals.

in chapter 2. Another might be the results of a doctor's examination. Yet a third could be your own self-analysis. Obviously the first two are more objective, but all are effective if they give you a clear idea of where you are starting from.

Step 2: Know where you want to go. Your goal will usually be based on a need or a desire. For example, your department or agency may have standards that you failed to meet on your assessment. Your doctor may tell you that you need to make lifestyle changes to avoid serious health problems. Or you may decide that you just want to look better.

Attaining any of these results may be your long-term goal, but it may take a while to get there. To avoid discouragement, you should set short-term goals. For example, you might set a goal of 10% improvement in fitness every 8 weeks until you reach the agency standard.

Make sure the goals you set are challenging, yet attainable (see Figure 13.1). If you were deficient on the 12-minute run, for example, planning to win next year's Boston Marathon is probably not a reasonable goal. In fact, if you are not sure how high to set

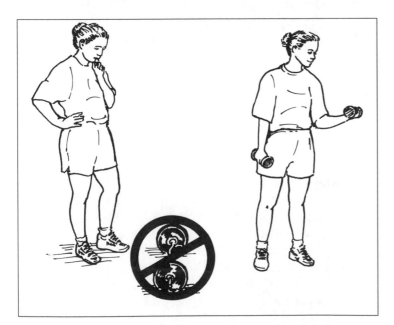

Figure 13.1 *While your goals should be challenging, they should also be realistic.*

your intermediate goals, it is probably better to set them a little too low than a little too high. While your goals should be challenging, it will be a more positive experience to reach the low goal than to fail on the high one. You can always readjust.

For many people, performance goals are more effective than outcome goals. For example, set your primary goal as exercising four times a week. Your secondary goal would be the improved scores on your assessment. This gives you greater control. You can guarantee that you will exercise four times a week, and if you do so you will almost certainly see the improvements you are striving for. But you have less control over the improvements.

Step 3: Decide what you need to do. This step links your goal setting with your program development, discussed in the preceding chapters. You should think through what you need to do in order to accomplish your goal. Make the goals specific. For example, to meet the agency's fitness standard, you will have to exercise at least three times a week. Following your doctor's orders may require changes in diet, smoking habits, or perhaps a combination of several things. Also take into consideration what resources you have to work with when setting your goals. For example, decide what will be the best time for exercise, what equipment you will need, and where you can find it.

Step 4: Check your progress. Obviously, to know if you are making progress you must periodically retest yourself. Set up a regular schedule to reevaluate yourself. For example, retesting every 4 weeks allows enough time for improvement between tests. You don't want to let too much time go by between tests so you can get a feel for the effectiveness of your program. If you do not see improvement after 4 weeks, especially early on, there is probably something lacking in your program. Most likely it is the intensity with which you are exercising.

If you fail to meet your goals at the end of the evaluation period, consider possible reasons. Did you exercise frequently enough, with the correct intensity, and for the prescribed time? If the answers to these questions are "yes," it's possible that you set your goals too high. Don't be discouraged.

As you learn more about your capabilities, you'll find that you can be more realistic in your goal setting. If you find after your first assessment that your initial goals were too high, adjusting them down to a more realistic level is not only acceptable but smart.

Goal setting is more effective when there are consequences for the outcomes, both positive and negative.

Determining Your Fitness Goals

You know what your scores are on each of the test items. But a test score (called a raw score) does not have any meaning by itself until it is compared to a norm or standard.

■ A norm indicates how one scored compared to a reference group. The reference group may be the general population or a group of similar age, gender, and/or occupation. For example, the norms shown in Table 2.3 (pp. 19-20) are grouped by age and gender.

■ A standard is a score point in the norms which has been defined as a performance criterion. For example, your agency may require you to score at the 50th percentile for each test item. That becomes the agency standard.

To get a good picture of how your scores compare with the norms, you can create a fitness profile, a chart that will show at a glance what areas you need to improve.

Fitness Profiling

In chapter 2, you compared your raw scores to a general index category of fitness. Now you will take that information and define specific goals for improvement, using your fitness profile. Figures 13.2 and 13.3 are provided for you to convert your raw scores to percentiles and to create your fitness profile. Take the following steps to create your fitness profile:

1. Write your raw scores for each event in the appropriate space on the Score Conversion Sheet.

Fitness area	Test	Raw Score	Percentile
Cardiovascular endurance (2 options)	$\dot{V}O_2$max	_____	_____
	12-min run	_____	_____
	1.5-mile run*	_____	_____
Flexibility	Sit-and-reach*	_____	_____
Muscular endurance	1-minute sit-up*	_____	_____
	Maximum push-up*	_____	_____
Muscular strength	1RM bench press	_____	_____
	1RM leg press	_____	_____
Body composition (3 options)	Skinfolds	_____	_____
	Circumference	_____	_____
	Body mass index	_____	_____
Anaerobic power	300-meter run	_____	_____

*Just indicate your scores for these four events if your agency does not administer a fitness test and you took the test in chapter 2.

Figure 13.2 *Score Conversion Sheet.*

2. Compare your raw scores to the age- and gender-adjusted norms in Table 2.3 (pp. 19-20).

3. Write the percentile for each event in the appropriate space.

4. On the Fitness Profile Sheet, place an "x" where your raw score falls for each event.

Just indicate your scores for these four events if your agency does not administer a fitness test and you took the test in chapter 2.

Sample Goal Setting

Take a look at how Officers Hernandez, Johnson, and Roberts approached their goal setting based on the results of their assessments.

Officer Hernandez

Officer Hernandez acknowledges he isn't very active. While he doesn't feel that he overeats, he does stop at the donut shop every day, and he recognizes that he eats a lot of sweets, has too much fat in his diet, and probably needs to lower his cholesterol. He has quit smoking, but stops off at the end of his

shift a few nights a week for a couple of beers with the boys. Tony usually gets 6 hours of fitful sleep a night. Of course he has stress on the job, and some at home, and there are days he feels that he is going to "blow his stack." His health and medical history is unremarkable except for his being overweight and getting no regular exercise.

Based on his physical fitness assessment, he needs to improve in most areas. He scored below the 5th percentile in aerobic fitness, leg press, and body composition; the 20th percentile for sit-ups; the 60th percentile for bench press; and the 30th percentile for flexibility. He didn't finish the 300-meter run. He was afraid it would kill him.

This is the same process you should go through at this point. There is no point in being anything less than 100% honest with yourself in any of the subjective evaluations. Remember, record all of your results, and see a doctor before continuing if you have any of the indicators outlined in chapter 2.

Tony knows that he must eventually meet the department's standard of being at the 50th percentile for aerobic fitness, strength, flexibility, 300-meter run, and body

	Anaerobic power Cardiovascular endurance		Flexibility	Muscular endurance		Muscular strength		Body composition
Fitness category	1.5-mile run*	300-m run	Sit-and-reach*	Sit-ups*	Push-ups*	Bench press	Leg press	% fat
Superior 95-100%								
Excellent 80-94%								
Good 60-79%								
Fair 40-59%								
Poor 20-39%								
Very poor 0-19%								

*Just indicate your scores for these four events if your agency does not administer a fitness test and you took the test in chapter 2.

Figure 13.3 *Fitness Profile Sheet.*

composition. Fortunately, they have given him adequate time to achieve the standards. He is motivated to make the lifestyle changes required and feels confident that he can meet the standards within the time limit. Through the department he has access to exercise equipment at the local community college. He has suggested to his wife that she should take an interest in fitness also. To be supportive and to improve her own fitness level, she has signed up for a continuing education module on basic fitness through the local parks and recreation program.

Based on his present condition, Tony will begin his aerobic training with a walking program. His goal is to walk 4 miles by the end of 8 weeks, and to improve his time on the 1.5-mile run to 16:30 by the end of 12 weeks. He recognizes that this may be very ambitious. His strength goals are to bench press 225 pounds, leg press 300 pounds, and do 27 sit-ups and 20 push-ups at the end of 8 weeks. He will begin and end each training session with 5 minutes of the stretching exercises shown in chapter 6, and he hopes to improve his score on the sit-and-reach test to 14 inches by that time. By combining exercise and diet, he plans to lose 15 pounds over the next 16 weeks, and lower his percent body fat to 27%. His goal for the 300-yard run is to run it in 80 seconds, but to finish it will be a good accomplishment.

His lifestyle goals will complement his exercise goals. Tony will limit his trips to the donut shop and the local watering hole to one a week. He will switch to light beer. Mrs. Hernandez will take some cooking classes to learn about preparing meals that are lower in fat, sodium, and cholesterol. She will buy frozen yogurt instead of ice cream, and pretzels instead of chips.

Tony has learned from the fitness spots on Law Enforcement Television Network that physical activity can reduce the negative effects of stress. If at the end of his first evaluation period he doesn't see any results, he will attend a stress management seminar sponsored by the department.

Officer Hernandez's goals are recorded in Figure 13.4.

Officer Johnson

Officer Johnson's needs are a little bit different. One of his biggest challenges is to quit smoking. His plan is to cut back gradually. One aspect of his plan is to stop taking work to the designated smoking area in the headquarters building. By restricting himself to his non-smoking office, Rosie figures that he can cut back his smoking by five packs a week. He'll use the money he saves to take his wife to a really nice restaurant each month.

While his department does not have a fitness program, Rosie wants to improve his physical conditioning. He scored well on the flexibility test, but was in the poor category on the 1.5-mile run and the sit-ups, and in the fair category for the push-ups. For the push-ups and sit-ups, he wants to improve to 25 and 37, respectively, in the next 8 weeks. He believes that he can improve to the fair category in the run within that time. His goal for the sit-and-reach is to improve by 1 inch.

Officer Roberts

Officer Roberts' department has mandatory testing but no standards. Therefore, much of her motivation for improvement is self-driven. Her assessment indicated that she is above average in all physical fitness categories except for strength. Her score on the bench press put her in the 10th percentile, and she was in the 30th percentile for the leg press. Even though Monique is not overweight, her cholesterol reading was 210, with an HDL of 39. She needs to be more careful about what she eats. When she evaluated her diet she saw that most of her fat intake came from saturated fats. She had thought that her diet was healthy because she ate a lot of chef salads, but she has now realized that the dressing, cold cuts, and cheese in the salads had been a major source of dietary fat.

Monique's goals are to improve to the 25th percentile in the bench press and to the 40th percentile in the leg press within 4 weeks. She also wants to improve her push-ups to 13 and her sit-ups to 30. She will have her cholesterol rechecked at that time, and will be satisfied if there is improvement.

While Monique's other physical measurements were satisfactory, she still wants to make improvements in some areas. She has established goals for modest improvements in the 1.5-mile run, 300-yard run, and body composition. Monique figures that the extra strength training she will be doing should add enough muscle to lower her percent body fat by 1%. By eliminating the cold cuts and cheeses from her salads, she will probably lower it even more.

Additional Sample Goals for Various Fitness Levels

Some of you may be interested in establishing goals that are beyond those connected to your agency's standards. For one thing, your agency is not likely to include behavioral goals like smoking cessation in their standards, but we know that healthy behaviors are an important part of overall fitness. You can use the personal inventory shown in Figure 13.5 to help you evaluate your lifestyle choices in light of your fitness goals. The following list will give you some more ideas for setting personal fitness goals.

1. For officers scoring at the 75th percentile and higher:
   a. Run a 10-km road race.
   b. Complete a half-marathon.
   c. Bench press 1.5 times your body weight.
   d. Participate in a triathlon.
2. For officers scoring between the 50th and 75th percentiles:

1. Cardiovascular endurance	Current raw score (min, sec)	17:54
	12-week goal	16:30
2. Flexibility	Current raw score (in.)	13
	8-week goal	14
3. Muscular endurance	Current raw score (number of sit-ups)	22
	8-week goal	27
	Current raw score (number of push-ups)	10
	8-week goal	20
4. Muscular strength	Current raw score (bench press lbs)	200
	8-week goal	225
	Current raw score (leg press lbs)	270
	8-week goal	300
5. Body composition	Current raw score (% fat or body mass index)	33% fat
	16-week goal	27%
	Current body weight (lbs)	230
	16-week goal body weight	215
6. Anaerobic power	Current raw score (sec)	---
	8-week goal	80 sec
7. Other goals		

Make only one trip to the donut shop each week.
Switch to light beer.
Eat frozen yogurt in place of ice cream.
Snack on pretzels instead of chips.

Figure 13.4 *Goal-setting sheet for Officer Hernandez.*

a. Complete a 5-km road race.

b. Bench press 1.25 times your body weight.

c. Reduce body fat by 3%.

d. Eliminate all "yes" responses on your personal inventory (Figure 13.5).

3. For officers scoring between the 25th and 50th percentiles:

   a. Establish a habit of working out at least three times a week for each component of fitness.

   b. Run 3 miles without undue fatigue.

   c. Bench press your body weight.

   d. Reduce percent body fat by 3%.

   e. Reduce the number of "yes" responses on your personal inventory by one each quarter (Figure 13.5).

4. For officers scoring below the 25th percentile:

   a. Establish a habit of working out three times a week for each component of fitness.

   b. Walk 3 miles without undue fatigue.

   c. Improve 1RM on each strength training exercise by 10% each quarter.

   d. Reduce percent body fat by 3%.

   e. Eliminate one "yes" response on your personal inventory each quarter (Figure 13.5).

Filling Out the Goal-Setting Worksheet

Now you should be ready to fill out the goal-setting worksheet shown in Figure 13.6. Follow the instructions given at the top of the worksheet.

Setting Goals

To set a goal for each fitness area, use the following information as a guide. Depending on your individual circumstances, you may want to set your goals higher or lower for each category.

■ If the fitness test raw score is at the *Good* category (60th percentile) or higher, then it is appropriate to maintain at that level. The goal would be to attain the same performance on subsequent tests.

■ If you are in the *Good* category or better, but still want to improve in one or more areas, multiply the raw score by .05 (5%). Subtract that number from the raw score for the 1.5-mile test, the 300-meter run, and the percent body fat. Add the 5% improvement number to the sit-and-reach, bench press, leg press, push-up, sit-up, and 12-minute run raw scores.

■ If the fitness test raw score is below the *Good* category, an improvement goal is appropriate. Multiply the raw score by .10 (10%). For each test item, add or subtract the improvement number as shown in the preceding paragraph.

■ For those who exercise regularly following the guidelines presented in chapters 4 through 7, it will take 3 to 4 weeks to achieve improvement in each component of fitness. Untrained persons may see some improvements in shorter times.

■ When setting time to achieve your goals, allow enough time to ensure that there will be some improvement, but don't set times so far out that you lose interest.

Answer "yes" or "no" to each of the following questions.	Yes	No
Do I need more exercise?	___	___
Would I like to look better?	___	___
Should I eat better?	___	___
Do I smoke?	___	___
Do I have more than two drinks per day?	___	___
Do I often experience stress?	___	___
Should I get more sleep?	___	___
Do I have other unhealthy behaviors?	___	___

Figure 13.5 *Personal inventory worksheet.*

Instructions: Fill in the appropriate blanks with your scores from the seven-item fitness assessment, or from the four-item test in chapter 2. Determine how much time you need to achieve your goal and enter the number of weeks in the corresponding blanks.

1. Aerobic power   Current raw score   _____
                                 (distance, time)

                                 _____ Week goal   _____

2. Flexibility   Current raw score (in.)   _____

                                 _____ Week goal   _____

3. Muscular endurance Current raw score   _____
                                 (number of sit-ups)

                                 _____ Week goal   _____

                                 Current raw score   _____
                                 (number of push-ups)

                                 _____ Week goal   _____

4. Absolute strength   Current raw score   _____
                                 (bench press ratio)

                                 _____ Week goal   _____

                                 Current raw score   _____
                                 (leg press ratio)

                                 _____ Week goal   _____

5. Body composition   Current raw score   _____
                                 (% fat or body mass index)

                                 _____ Week goal   _____

                                 Current body weight (lbs) _____

                                 _____ Week goal   _____
                                 body weight

6. Anaerobic power   Current raw score (time)   _____

                                 _____ Week goal   _____

7. Other goals

   a. Smoking cessation

   b. Stress management

   c. Control of substance abuse

Figure 13.6 *Goal-setting sheet.*

- Allowing from 4 to 12 weeks between retests should accomplish your objective. Of course this will depend upon factors such as your work schedule, how faithful you are to your workout schedule, and injuries.

Goal-Setting Steps

To fill out the goal-setting sheet, follow these steps:

1. Make several copies of the worksheet because you will periodically reassess your goals.

2. From your assessment sheet, fill in the scores on each of the tests.

3. Once you have decided on a goal for each of the events, record it in the last column.

4. Decide on how much time you are going to give yourself to achieve each goal, and record it in the appropriate space. Remember the guidelines on how long it takes to achieve a training effect, and time your goal accordingly.

5. Under "Other goals," enter your non-physical fitness goals. Be specific. For example, lower your cholesterol, quit smoking, or lose 15 pounds.

6. Post a copy of your goals where you will see them several times every day. Make sure that you have a copy of your diet goals visible in the kitchen.

Goal setting is important in everything that you do. It's virtually impossible to accomplish anything worthwhile if you do not know what it is you are trying to achieve. Use the information here and in the next chapter to give yourself a realistic road map to get you where you want to go, and an idea of what roadblocks may get in your way.

CHAPTER 14

Realistic Expectations

Officer Hernandez really did want to lose weight and get into shape. He learned about exercise and the lifestyle changes that he needed to make. He set his goals and started his program with high expectations. The first 2 weeks went pretty well. He missed only one exercise session and did well with his new eating plan. According to the scale he lost 4 pounds, although he couldn't see any change himself. The third week he stopped at the donut shop twice, and was slipping up on his other eating promises. The fourth week was really busy, and he got out to walk only one time. His wife was trying hard to encourage him. Tony perceived her words as nagging and began stopping off for a beer after shift each night. Before he knew it, he was right back where he had started. Tony asked himself if it was worth it. He decided that maybe he just didn't have the self-discipline necessary to change his habits.

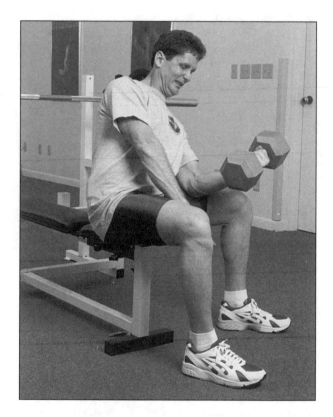

When you finish this chapter, you will be able to:

- ✪ Recognize the signs that you are losing motivation.
- ✪ Know the predictors of dropping out.
- ✪ Understand the times you are most likely to slip from a program.
- ✪ Take actions to avoid becoming a drop-out.
- ✪ Get back on track after a lapse or drop-out.

Officer Roberts, on the other hand, was still on her program 6 weeks later. She was in the weight room three or four times each week and was finding it relatively easy to stay with her new eating plan. After 6 weeks, her strength had improved and her total cholesterol was down to 202. These improvements inspired her to work even harder.

Results like these are not uncommon and could possibly even have been predicted. In this chapter, you'll learn about expectations, predictors of who is likely to drop out of a fitness program, and some ways to avoid being a fitness drop-out.

What Is the Extent of the Problem?

Is Officer Hernandez or Officer Roberts typical when it comes to sticking with an exercise program? Here are some statistics that will help you see the extent of the problem.

- Exercise

    - 50% drop out within 6 months to a year

    - 75% drop out within 3 years

- Eating habits

    - 20% to 80% fail to follow a prescribed diet

    - 90% fail to reach weight-loss goals

- Smoking

    - 60% to 90% go back to smoking within 6 months

    It appears that Officer Hernandez, on the verge of becoming a fitness drop-out, is typical of people trying to change their lifestyles. Could his potential for dropping out have been predicted?

Predictors of Exercise Program Quitters

Behavioral scientists have been intrigued with the problem of sticking to exercise programs, and have identified some common denominators among fitness drop-outs. They have categorized these characteristics as psychological, behavioral, biological, social/ environmental, and programming. These characteristics are listed in Table 14.1. You can see from this table that Officer Hernandez's inability to stick with the program is predictable. Having low self-esteem, he didn't expect to be successful. His previous inactive lifestyle, low fitness level, and high body fat are other factors working against him. However, he does have some favorable existing items listed under the social/environmental and programming factors. As you will see, all is not lost for Officer Hernandez.

You might suspect that Officer Roberts would stick to her program. Already fit, she is used to disciplining herself to stay with an exercise regime. Because she doesn't have as many lifestyle changes to make, she can concentrate more effort on those that need work. She is seeing results, which further encourages her to stay with the changes in her behavior.

Look at the factors in Table 14.1 and decide if you are potentially a fitness dropout. Your attitude shouldn't be that you can't overcome these obstacles. Rather, you need to be aware that sticking with the program may be tougher for you, and you must commit yourself to extra effort if you are to be successful.

Studies conducted to examine this issue have identified reasons given by those who stick with exercise and those who drop out. Table 14.2 presents these reasons.

While Tony may agree with every reason given in the first column, the second column more closely describes his status. Finding time may seem to be a problem for all law enforcement officers, especially before fitness becomes a lifestyle. He obviously doesn't have a very good attitude about fitness or he wouldn't have let himself get so far out of condition. He may feel now that he can never recover. It can be easy to get discouraged when you don't see results as quickly as you may like.

Dangerous Times

You should know that there are three dangerous times for potentially dropping out of your program: after the assessment, after two or three sessions, and after completing a formal program.

After the Assessment

You may feel that you are too far out of shape to make the effort worthwhile. Remember why you wanted to get started in the first place. Also remember the old Chinese proverb that "a journey of a thousand miles begins with a single step."

Table 14.1
Factors Predicting Drop-Outs

Psychological factors		Behavioral factors	Biological factors
Low self-esteem	Apathy	Inactive lifestyle	Low fitness level
High depression	Low willpower	Smoker	High body fat
High anxiety	Low persistence	Type A person	Injury prone
High extroversion	Low dependability	Always rushed	
Low expectancy of success	Low determination	Poor credit	
Lack of self-motivation	Low organization	Lack of ability to set goals	
Social/environmental factors		**Programming factors**	
Low family support		Inconvenient	Too costly
Low peer support		Lack of leader modeling	Lack of information
Lack of leadership		Lack of feedback and reinforcement	Lack of structure
Lack of cultural support		Inflexible goals	
Lack of group activity support		Too high an activity intensity	
Lack of organizational support		Lack of individual prescription	
Type of job situation: high travel, change		Lack of activity variety	

Table 14.2
Differences Between Exercisers and Drop-Outs

Why adults say they exercise	Why adults say they drop out	
Health	No interest	No time
Look good	Poor choice of program or facilities	No energy
Be with a group	Competing health-compromising lifestyles	Too far out of shape
Feel good	Poor perception of and attitude about exercise	No results
Minimize aging	Poor choice of exercise mode	Don't know how to get started
Have fun	Pre-existing injury or illness	

After Two Sessions

The first few exercise sessions may be a serious shock to your body. After perhaps years of inactivity, suddenly stressing the body can result in pain and soreness. You have to resist the temptation to do too much too soon.

After Completing a Formal Program

During a formal program, you will have support and incentives that may not exist when you are on your own. The loss of these when the program ends can be daunting, but don't let it scare you away from continuing toward your goal of a fitter, healthier you.

Dropping Out

There are usually two levels of setbacks before you become a drop-out. Understanding what they are and how they relate to dropping out can help you avoid discouragement.

Slips

Everyone has some slips in her or his program. A slip is not a failure. Slips may come from unavoidable circumstances or from laziness. In either case, while it's important to stick to your goal, recognize that a slip does not sabotage your effort. If you can make it up, do it. If not, don't think that your conditioning has been affected so seriously that further effort is useless. Just don't let your slips progress into a lapse.

Lapses

When do slips become a lapse? A lapse represents a return to your former unwanted behaviors. If you have gone more than a week without exercising, for example, you may consider yourself to have suffered a lapse. While clearly more serious than a slip, a lapse is not the end of the world either. Once again, remind yourself of why you started the program, and how good you will feel when you have reached your goals. Get back on track as soon as possible to avoid becoming a fitness drop-out.

Drop-Outs

When you have dropped out, it means that you have abandoned your program. You have decided that you can't do it, and your goals aren't important enough for you to make the trade-offs necessary to accomplish them.

How to Avoid Slippage Problems

Everyone has bad days and sometimes needs a little extra push to get out of the door for exercise. Now you'll learn some ideas on how to avoid being a dropout statistic.

External Versus Internal Motivation

Think back to why you decided to start a fitness program and recall the reasons you did so. Chances are there were a number of reasons, but try to decide which was the most important one. Was it because you were concerned about the consequences of not meeting the agency's standards? If so, your strongest motivation was external.

On the other hand, if you decided to start a fitness program because you wanted to perform better, or to look better, or for any other reason that was driven by your own needs or wants, then your motivation is internal.

Research has shown that internal motivators are stronger. You are more likely to stick with it when you are doing something for reasons that you have decided are important. If you haven't identified any internal motivators for undertaking a fitness program up until now, it would be a good idea to do so.

Positive Thinking

Think in terms of "when," not "if," goals will be attained. We hear and read all of the time about the power of positive thinking, and there is definitely some truth to the concept that thinking positively can help reach goals. Having doubts about your ability to achieve your goals is a defeatist attitude and can only increase the chances of not meeting them.

Practice

It takes a minimum of 3 to 4 weeks for habits to form. Practicing your new behaviors regularly is the only way to make them become the habits that you want them to be. The other element besides regularity that's important is correctness. Practicing a new behavior incorrectly is counter-productive.

Supervision

Even professional athletes have coaches. Besides helping them to identify and correct inappropriate behaviors, coaches help keep their athletes on the right track. Your "coach" could be your agency's fitness coordinator, your partner, or anyone else who wants to help you stay on track.

Planning

You already know that planning can make the difference in most everything you do. There is an old adage that says, "Failing to plan is the same as planning to fail." If you take a haphazard approach to your training, you may not even know if you are falling short of the required number of training sessions per week, because you won't have a yardstick to compare your efforts against. Set up your training schedule at least 1 week in advance and don't let anything short of a catastrophe get in your way of sticking with it.

Realistic Expectations

Know that some days will be tougher than others. Doing something on those bad days is better than not doing anything. You'll also often find that once you get started you'll feel better than you thought you would, and you can get the work done that you planned on. Also remember that slips are not failures.

Progress

Keep heading in the direction of your goals. While you're going to have bad days, you can overcome them. If your goals are important enough to you, nothing can stop you except yourself.

Ways to Improve Your Own Perseverance

In addition to avoiding problems, you can further strengthen your commitment to your program by some of the positive actions listed here.

Join Groups

There are several reasons why joining a group can help you stick with a program. For many people, the social aspect of exercising with a group is appealing. Others will feel as though they are letting the group down if they miss an exercise session. In addition to getting an individual to show up, the group is also like-ly to make the person give a better effort during the exercise session itself.

Plan Exercise With Family and Friends

Some of the benefits of this approach are the same as joining a group. The added benefits of exercising with family and friends are that they are familiar to you and interested in your success. You may feel more comfortable exercising with people that you know well. For their part, they may be more likely to encourage your continued participation than would a group of strangers.

Learn About Healthy Lifestyle Choices

The more you know about a subject, the more you are likely to make correct choices. The more your understanding of the benefits of exercise and other healthy lifestyle choices increases, the more you will want to stay with a program that will give you improvements in performance and health.

Reward Yourself

Most experts agree that having consequences for your actions is an effective way to ensure that you will maintain a new behavior. Likewise, they agree that rewards are better motivators than are punishments. Simple rewards along the way can help you stay with the program. Identify what it is you like to do, whom you like to be with, where you like to go, and then build your reward system around these ideas. One word of caution—don't make the reward self-defeating. For example, don't reward yourself for losing 10 pounds by eating a banana split.

Enlist a Helper

Ask your partner, a spouse, or a friend to help you attain your goals. Explain to them how important it is to you and give them some ways that they can help you. For example, they might call you 30 minutes before your workout time each day as a reminder. They

I will:

Walk five times a week until I can go 4 miles without undue fatigue.

Do my strength training three times a week. If I can't get to the fitness center, I will substitute the calisthenic circuit.

Improve my 1RM by 10% in 8 weeks.

Stretch for 5 minutes before and after each workout.

Limit my trips to the donut shop to one a week.

Substitute pretzels for chips, and yogurt for ice cream.

Lose 8 pounds in the next 8 weeks.

I will enlist the help of:

My wife

My partner

My responsibilities:

Schedule my fitness activities for 4 weeks out, and update my schedule every Sunday.

Coordinate my schedule with my wife and my partner.

Maintain a log of my activities and my eating habits.

My helpers' responsibilities:

Remind me 1 hour before my scheduled activities.

Harass me if I miss a workout.

My wife will prepare low-fat, low-cholesterol meals. Replace chips and ice cream with pretzels and yogurt.

Provide encouragement and support.

My reward:

New pair of running shoes when I attain my walking goal.

Tickets for ballgame for 8 consecutive weeks of perfect attendance.

New clothes for losing 8 pounds.

My consequence for falling short of my goal:

Putting my picture with the word Quitter under it on the office bulletin board.

Date: 12/4/94

   Participant: Tony Hernandez

   Helper: Angelica Hernandez

   Partner: Alan Ruddy

Figure 14.1 *Officer Hernandez's fitness contract.*

may even choose to exercise with you. There are also some things you may ask them not to do. For example, they can help you by not tempting you with food when you are trying to lose weight. A technique for utilizing a helper is to make a fitness contract.

Making a Contract

As noted earlier, having your goals in writing may improve your ability to stay with the program. Some people use a contract to further solidify their commitment.

After reading this chapter and analyzing his situation, Officer Hernandez decided that making a contract would get him back on track, and improve his motivation when he restarted his fitness program. Figure 14.1 shows how Officer Hernandez filled out his fitness contract. Figure 14.2 shows a sample contract that you may want to use.

You know that it is important for law enforcement officers to be fit. You also know the health risks associated with the lack of a total fitness program. You have the information you need to successfully undertake a fitness program which will improve your health and performance. You have learned how to set goals, how to adjust them, and how to improve your motivation. Put it all together and add the last critical ingredient—your commitment to improved health and performance. With that ingredient, you will be on the road to a longer, healthier life—during the rest of your career and as you enjoy the fruits of your labor during retirement.

Suggested Readings

Dishman, R.K. (Ed.) (1988). *Exercise adherence: Its impact on public health.* Champaign, IL: Human Kinetics.

Roberts, G.C. (Ed.) (1992). *Motivation in sport and exercise.* Champaign, IL: Human Kinetics.

Willis, J.D., & Campbell, L.F. (1992). *Exercise psychology.* Champaign, IL: Human Kinetics.

I will:

_____

_____

_____

_____

_____

_____

_____

I will enlist the help of:

_____

_____

My responsibilities:

_____

_____

_____

My helpers' responsibilities:

_____

_____

_____

_____

My reward:

_____

_____

_____

My consequence for falling short of my goal:

_____

_____

Date: _____

   Participant: _____

   Helper: _____

   Partner: _____

Figure 14.2 *Fitness contract.*

Weight Training Exercises

The following exercise descriptions correspond to the exercises listed in Table 5.2 (p. 44). Only the free weight exercises are illustrated here because the wide variation in exercise machines available would make it difficult to illustrate every variation possible.

Heel Raises With Weight on Back

Place the bar on your shoulders and stand on an elevated, stable surface approximately 6 inches high. Place your feet hip-width apart with the balls of both feet near the edge. You may vary your feet from straight ahead to slightly outward to inward. Keep your torso erect and knees straight.

Slowly raise your heels as high as possible. Pause momentarily before lowering, allowing only your calves to do the work. Exhale as you ascend.

Slowly lower your heels to a full stretch without pain. Do not move your torso or flex your knees. Inhale as you descend.

Half-Knee Bends (or Squats) With Weight on Back

Use an overhand grip, slightly wider than shoulder width, and place the bar on your shoulders at the base of your neck. Keep your torso and hips directly under the bar with your chest out, shoulders back, and head up. Your feet should be flat on the

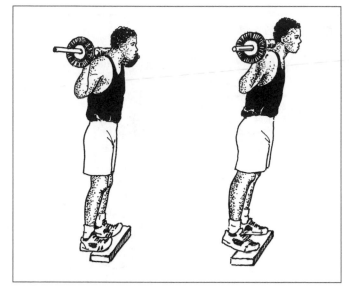

Heel Raises

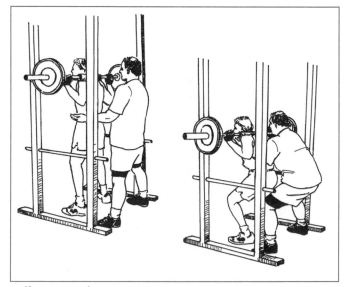

Half-Knee Bends

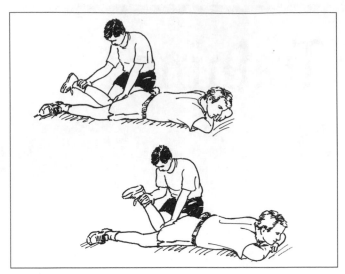

Leg Flexion

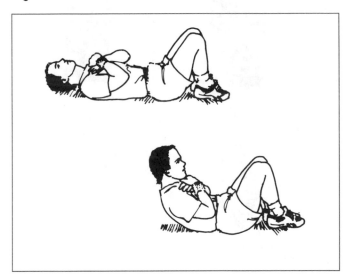

Sit-Ups

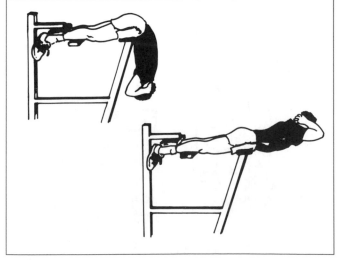

Trunk Lifts

floor, slightly wider than shoulder width. A spotter should stand directly behind you, keeping his or her back flat and knees flexed. Throughout the rest of the exercise, the spotter's hands should stay close to the bar and follow it during the lift.

Squat down slowly, inhaling as you descend. Avoid leaning forward excessively and keep your feet flat on the floor with your knees in line with your feet. Squat until the bottoms of your thighs are parallel to the floor.

Begin the upward movement with your legs first, keeping your head up and chest out. Straighten your hips and knees and exhale as you do so.

Leg Flexion

You'll need a partner for this exercise. Lie face down with your legs extended. Flex one leg against your partner's resistance until your heel is as close to your buttocks as possible. Next, resist your partner's efforts as he or she returns you to the starting position. Repeat this exercise with the other leg.

Sit-Ups

Lie with your back and feet flat on the floor and knees flexed at 90°. Fold your arms across your chest. If necessary, anchor your feet under a couch, or have a partner hold them. Curl your chin to your chest first and then raise your shoulders and upper back to a 30° to 45° angle, exhaling as you sit up. Pause in this position and then slowly return to the starting position, inhaling as you move down. Keep your chin to your chest until your shoulders touch the mat and then lower your head. Pause in this position before beginning another repetition.

Trunk Lifts

Lie face down on a hyperextension bench with your knees level with your hips. The pads should be in contact with your hips and the backs of your ankles. Hang your torso down to form a 90° angle at the hip. Place your hands on each side of your head or crossed at the chest.

Raise your trunk until your upper torso is parallel to the floor. Your head should face forward and your thighs and shoulders should form a straight line. Exhale through the upward movement. Inhale as you lower your upper body slowly to return to the beginning position.

Bench Press

Use an overhand grip with your hands at least shoulder-width apart. Position your body so that you have four points of contact—your head, shoulders, and buttocks on the bench and your feet on the floor. The spotter should position his or her feet 2 to 6 inches from the bench and use an alternate grip inside your hands.

Signal the spotter to assist you in moving the bar off the supports. Push the bar to a straight-elbow position over your chest. The spotter should assist with moving the bar off the supports and guide the bar to the straight-elbow position. Throughout the rest of the exercise, the spotter's hands should closely follow the bar movement, ready to assist if necessary.

Inhale as you lower the bar slowly to your chest. Keep your wrists straight and directly above your elbows. Exhale as you push the bar upward under control. Your elbows should extend evenly and your wrists should be directly above your elbows. Pause at the straight-elbow position.

Bent Rowing

Use an overhand grip with hands at least shoulder-width apart and shoulders higher than hips. Your lower back should be flat, your elbows straight, your head facing forward, and your knees slightly flexed.

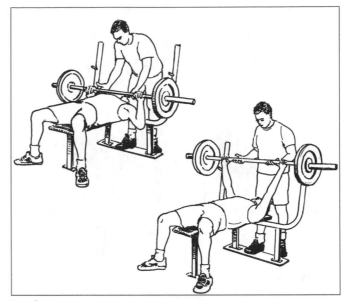

Bench Press

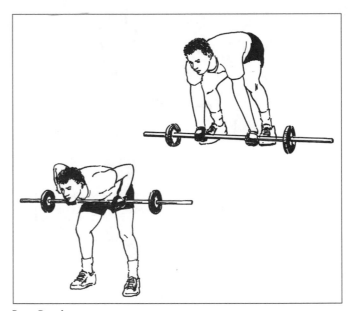

Bent Rowing

Slowly pull the bar straight up and pause momentarily before it touches your chest. Keep your torso rigid and exhale as the bar nears your chest. Inhale as you slowly lower the bar straight down, being careful not to bounce or jerk the bar at the bottom. Do not allow the bar to touch the floor until the set is complete.

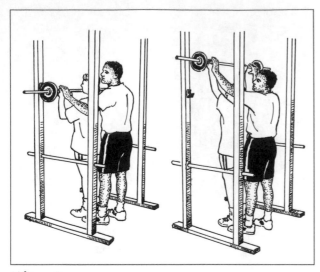

Military Press

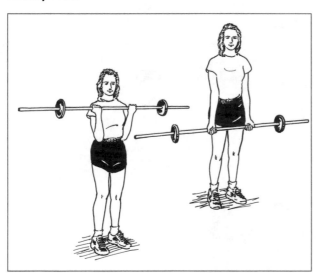

Biceps Curls

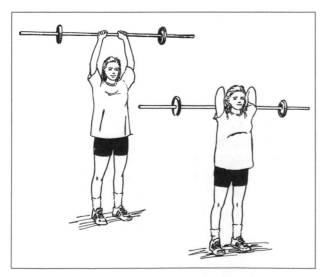

Triceps Extension

Military Press

Use an overhand grip, evenly spaced, with your hands at least shoulder-width apart. Keep your head upright and facing forward and keep your elbows under the bar with wrists extended. The bar should rest in your hands and on your shoulders. A spotter should stand as close as possible directly behind you, feet shoulder-width apart. Throughout the rest of the exercise, the spotter's hands should follow the bar closely.

Push the bar straight up while your back remains flat and erect. Exhale through the sticking point and pause at the top of the movement. Lower the bar slowly while inhaling. Do not bounce the bar off your upper chest.

Biceps Curls

Use an underhand grip with hands shoulder-width apart. The bar should touch the front of your thighs. Your upper arms should be against your ribs, your elbows extended, your torso erect, and your head facing forward.

Keep your upper arms stationary and your elbows close to your body as you curl the bar to your shoulders. Be careful not to rock, jerk, or swing your body as you lift. Exhale as the bar nears your shoulders. Inhale during the downward movement, lowering the bar slowly to your thighs. Keep your elbows close to your sides and extend your arms completely.

Triceps Extension

Use an overhand grip with hands 6 inches apart. Keep your torso erect, your head facing forward, your feet shoulder-width apart, and your fully extended elbows close to your ears.

Inhale as you lower the bar behind your head to the top of your shoulders. Keep your elbows pointed up and control the downward movement of the bar. Then push the bar until your elbows are again fully extended. Keep your elbows back and close to your ears. Exhale as the bar passes through the sticking point.

Static Stretching Exercises

The following static stretch descriptions correspond to the stretches listed in Figure 6.2 on p. 52. All the stretches described here are important, but some are absolutely essential. For a list of the 10 stretches that are considered to be essential, refer to Figure 6.3 on p. 52.

Ankles

Sit upright with one leg crossed over the opposite knee. Hold above your ankle with one hand and grasp the top portion of your foot with the other hand. Exhale and slowly pull the bottom of your foot to your body. Hold and relax.

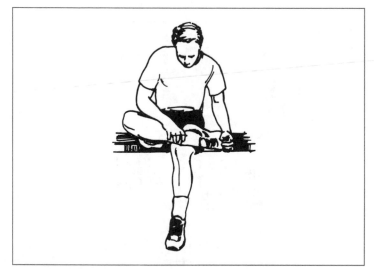

Ankles

Lower Leg

Sit upright on the floor with one leg straight and the other positioned so that its heel touches the opposite thigh. Exhale, bend forward at the waist, and grasp your foot. Exhale and slowly turn your ankle inward. Hold and relax.

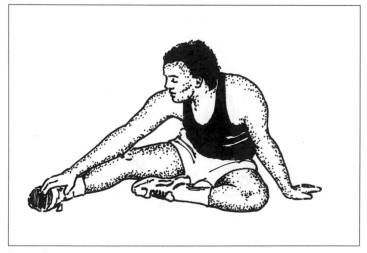

Lower Leg

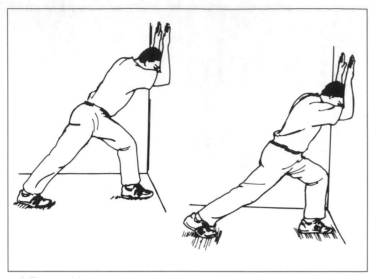

Achilles Tendon

Achilles Tendon

Stand upright four or five steps from a wall. Bend one leg forward and keep your opposite leg straight. Lean against the wall while keeping your body in a straight line and your rear foot flat and parallel to your hips. Exhale, bend your arms, move your chest toward the wall, and shift your weight forward. Hold and relax. You can also perform this stretch keeping your heel raised until you shift your weight forward, then try to lower your rear heel to the floor while exhaling.

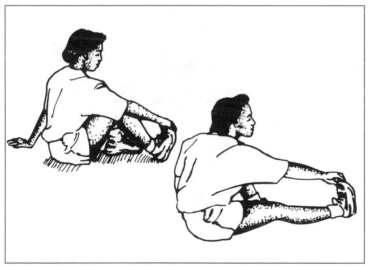

Back of Knee

Back of Knee

Sit upright on the floor with your knees flexed and grasp the toes of one foot. Exhale and slowly extend the leg. Exhale and pull back on the foot. Hold and relax.

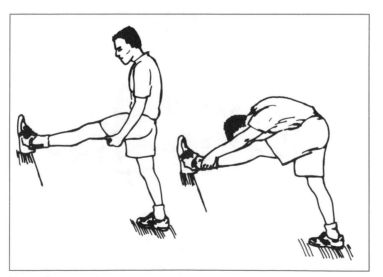

Hamstrings

Hamstrings

Stand upright, slowly raise one leg, and rest it on an elevated platform at a comfortable height. Exhale, keep both legs straight and your hips squared, extend your upper back, bend forward at the waist, and lower your trunk onto your raised thigh. Hold and relax.

Quadriceps

Lie face down with your body extended. Flex one leg and bring your heel toward your buttocks. Exhale, swing your arm back to grasp your ankle, and pull your heel toward your buttocks without over-compressing the knee. Hold and relax.

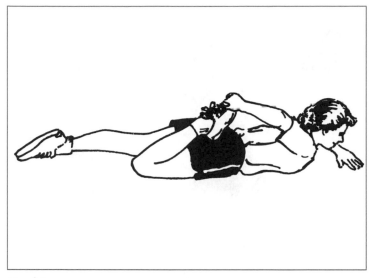

Quadriceps

Groin

Sit upright on the floor. Flex your knees and bring the heels and soles of your feet together as you pull them toward your buttocks. Place your elbows on the inside portion of both upper legs. Exhale and slowly push your legs to the floor. Hold and relax.

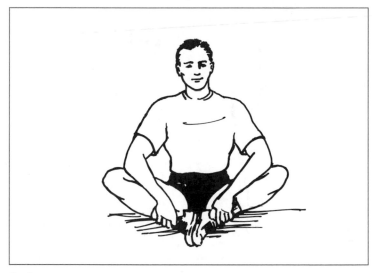

Groin

Hip Flexors

Stand upright with the legs strad-dled 2 feet apart. Turn your right foot 90° sideways to the right, keeping your toes and heel in line with your body. Flex your right knee and roll your left foot under so the top of the instep rests on the floor. Place your hands on your hips. Exhale and slowly lean or push your left hip toward the floor. Hold and relax.

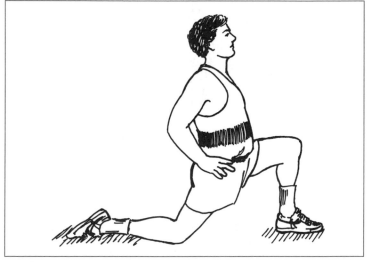

Hip Flexors

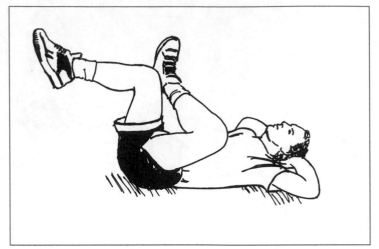

Buttocks

Buttocks

Lie flat on your back with your left leg crossed over your right knee. Inhale, flex your right knee, and let it push your left foot toward your face while keeping your head, shoulders, and back flat on the floor. Hold and relax.

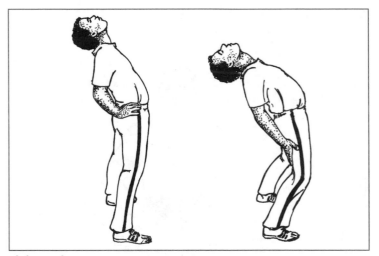

Abdominals

Abdominals

Stand upright with legs straddled 2 or 3 feet apart and hands placed on hips. Exhale, slowly arch your back, contract your buttocks, and push your hips forward. Exhale, continue arching your back, drop your head backward, and gradually slide your hands below your buttocks. Hold and relax.

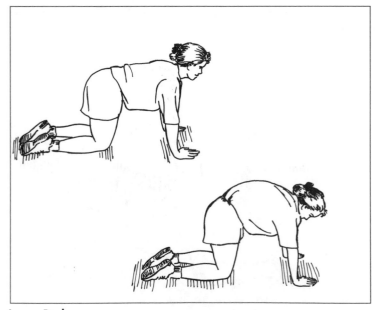

Lower Back

Lower Back

Kneel on all fours with your toes facing backward and your back flat. Inhale, contract your abdominals, and round your back. Exhale, relax your abdominals, and return to the flat-back position.

Trunk

Sit upright on the floor with your legs crossed. Interlock your hands behind your head with the elbows lifted. Exhale, bring your right elbow to your right knee, and keep your left shoulder and elbow back. Hold and relax.

Upper Back

Kneel on all fours. Extend your arms forward and lower your chest toward the floor. Exhale, extend your shoulders, and press down on the floor with your arms to produce an arch in your back. Hold and relax.

Neck

(a) Lie flat on the floor with both knees flexed. Interlock your hands on the back of your head near the crown. Exhale and pull your head off the floor and onto your chest. Keep your shoulder blades flat on the floor. Hold and relax.

(b) Sit or stand upright. Place your left hand on the upper right side of your head. Exhale and slowly pull the left side of your head onto your left shoulder. Hold and relax.

(c) Lie flat on a table with your head hanging over the edge. Hold and relax.

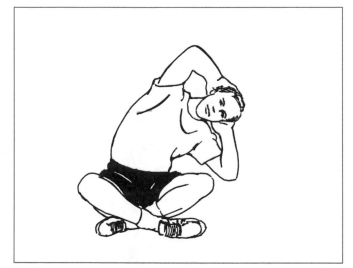

Trunk

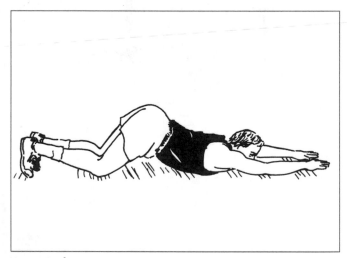

Upper Back

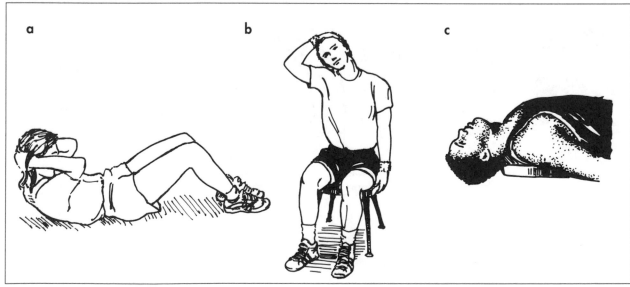

Neck

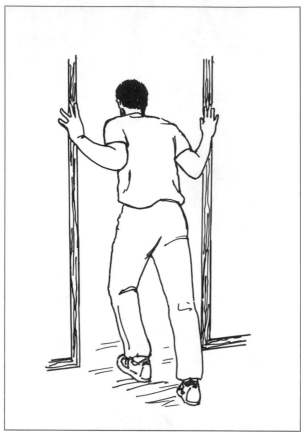

Pectorals

Pectorals

Stand upright facing a corner or open doorway. Raise your arms in a reverse "T" (elbows below your shoulders) and put your hands on the wall or the door jambs. Exhale and lean your entire body forward. Hold and relax.

Shoulders

(a) Sit upright on the floor with your hands about 1 foot behind your hips, your fingers pointing away from your body, and your legs extended forward. Inhale, lift your buttocks, raise your trunk off the floor, and open your chest as wide as possible. Hold and relax.

(b) Sit with one arm raised to shoulder height. Flex your arm across to the opposite shoulder. Grasp your raised elbow with the opposite hand. Exhale and pull your elbow backward. Hold and relax.

(c) Sit or stand upright with one arm flexed behind your back. Grasp the elbow from behind with the opposite hand. Exhale and pull your elbow across the midline of your back. Hold and relax.

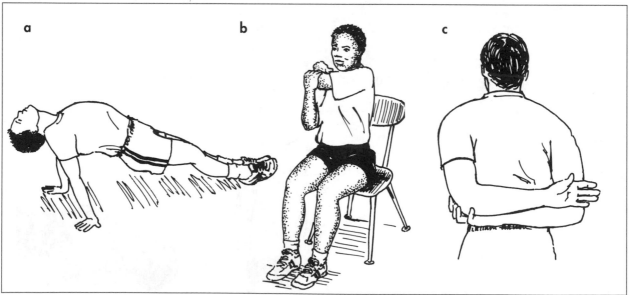

Shoulders

Biceps

Stand upright with your back to a doorframe. Rest one hand against the doorframe with your arm externally rotated at the shoulder, your forearm extended, and your hand pronated with your thumb pointing down. Exhale and attempt to roll your biceps so that they face upward. Hold and relax.

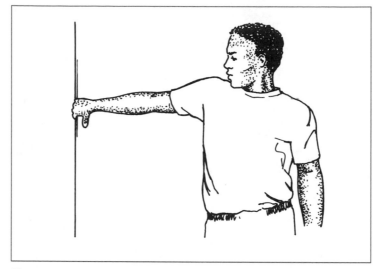

Biceps

Triceps

Flex one arm, raise it overhead next to your ear, and rest the hand on your shoulder blade. Grasp the elbow with the opposite hand. Exhale and pull your elbow behind your head. Hold and relax.

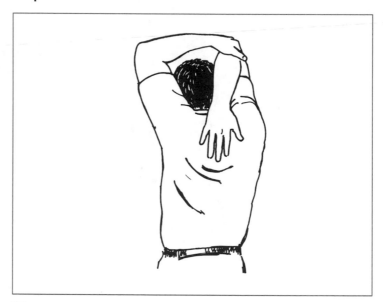

Triceps

Professional Support Organizations

American Cancer Society
777 Third Avenue
New York, NY 10017
800-227-2345

American Heart Association
7320 Greenville Avenue
Dallas, TX 75231
214-373-6300

American Hospital
Association
840 N. Lakeshore Dr.
Chicago, IL 60611
312-280-6000

American Lung Association
1740 Broadway
New York, NY 10019
212-315-8700

Business Health Education
Programs
Division of Northern
California Research
965 Mission St., Ste. 750
San Francisco, CA 94103
415-777-0611

Canadian Cancer Society
10 Alcorn Ave., Ste. 200
Toronto, ON M4V 3B1
416-961-7223

Canadian Heart and Stroke
Foundation
160 George St., Ste. 200
Ottawa, ON K1N 9M2
613-241-4361

Canadian Lung Association
1900 City Park Dr., Ste. 508
Gloucester, ON K1J 1A3
613-747-6776

Cardio-Fitness Center
345 Park Ave.
New York, NY 10022
212-838-4570

Center for Health Promotion
Health Central, Inc.
2810 57th Ave. N
Minneapolis, MN 55430
612-574-7800

Cooper Institute for Aerobics
Research
12330 Preston Road
Dallas, TX 75230
214-701-8001

Diabetic Athletes Association
1931 East Rovey Avenue
Phoenix, AZ 85016
602-433-2113

Executive Fitness Center
3 World Trade Center
New York, NY 10048
212-466-9266

Health & Human Resources
Group
922 Pennsylvania Ave. SE
Washington, DC 20003
202-727-2832

Health Mangement Associates
2120 S. Ash St.
Denver, CO 80222
303-692-0767

National Heart, Lung and
Blood Institute
Building 31, Room 4A-21
National Institutes of Health
Bethesda, MD 20205
301-957-3260

Office on Smoking and Health
158 Park Building
5600 Fishers Lande
Rockville, MD 20857
404-488-5705

Index

A

Absenteeism rates, 10
Achilles tendon stretch (exercise), 116
ACSM (American College of Sports Medicine), 12-13
Adaptation principle, 24
Abdominal muscle stretch (exercise), 118
Aerobic power. *See* Cardiovascular endurance
Air pollution, and training, 35-36
Alcohol abuse
  consequences of, 7, 87, 88-89
  statistics on, 7, 88
  stress and, 8, 76
  treatment for, 89
Alcoholic beverage consumption guidelines, 64, 67, 89. *See also* Alcohol abuse
Altitude, and training, 34-35
American College of Sports Medicine (ACSM), 12-13
American Institute of Stress, 60
Anabolic steroid use, 7, 87, 90
Anaerobic fitness/power, 55-60
  definition of, 4, 55
  law enforcement requirements for, 56
  program for developing, 56-58
Ankle stretch (exercise), 115
Assessment. *See* Fitness testing; Progress checks; Screening

B

Back of knee stretch (exercise), 116
Back pain, 6, 7, 15, 76
Back stretches (exercises), 118, 119
Balance principle
  definition of, 26
  for flexibility training, 53
  for resistance training, 42-43
Ballistic stretching, 51
Bench press (exercise), 43, 113
Bent rowing (exercise), 43, 46, 113
Biceps curls (exercise), 43, 114
Biceps stretch (exercise), 121
Blood pressure. *See also* High blood pressure
  resistance training and, 38
  screening test for, 14
BMI. *See* Body mass index calculation
Body composition. *See also* Obesity; Weight management
  assessment of, 71-72
  current levels among officers, 8
  definition of, 5
  guidelines for, 70
Body mass index calculation, 72. *See also* Body composition
Body weight, screening test for, 14. *See also* Obesity; Weight management
Borg, Gunnar, 32, 33
Breast cancer, 7
Bronchitis, 7, 81, 83
Buttocks stretch (exercise), 118

C

Caffeinated beverage consumption guidelines, 64, 67
Calcium, 7, 65
California Peace Officers Association, 9
Calisthenic training program, 45-47
Cancer
  body composition and, 70
  breast cancer, 7
  causes of, 7, 81, 82, 89
  colon cancer, 7
  lung cancer, 6, 7, 81, 82, 83
  mortality statistics, 6, 82
  nutrition and, 67
Carbohydrates, 62
Carbon monoxide, 36
Cardiorespiratory endurance. *See* Cardiovascular endurance
Cardiovascular disease
  benefits of exercise for, 10
  benefits of smoking cessation for, 83
  causes of, 7, 70, 76, 81, 82
  mortality statistics, 6, 81
  precautions with resistance training, 38
  screening for risk of, 12-13
Cardiovascular endurance (CVE, cardiorespiratory endurance, stamina), 29-36
  body composition and, 70
  current levels among officers, 8

definition of, 4, 30
fitness tests for, 16-18
law enforcement require-
    ments for, 4, 5, 30
physiological processes for,
    29
training program for, 30-36
Carrying, skill level required
    for, 5
Chair dips (exercise), 46
Chin-ups (exercise), 46
Cholesterol
    body composition and, 70
    in cardiovascular disease
        risk, 62, 82
    nutrition and, 62-63, 66
    screening test for, 14
Cigarette smoking. *See*
    Smoking; Smoking cessa-
    tion
Climbing, skill level required
    for, 5
Coaches, and motivation, 106
Cold weather, training in, 34, 35
Colon cancer, 7
Commission on Accreditation of
    Law Enforcement
    Agencies, 9
Contractions, muscle, 38
Contracts, fitness, 108, 109
Conversion of scores, 97-98
Cool-downs, 54
Cooper Institute for Aerobics
    Research, 8, 9
Cooper Test, 13
Coronary risk factors, screening
    for, 12-13. *See also*
    Cardiovascular disease
Costs of health care, 6, 7, 10, 81
Curls (exercises), 43, 46, 114
CVE. *See* Cardiovascular
    endurance

D

Death rates, 6, 7, 9, 81, 82, 83
Design of programs. *See* Fitness
    program design
Diabetes, 7, 67, 70
Diet. *See* Nutrition
Dieting, 70-71. *See also* Weight
    management
Disability, 9, 10

Disease. *See also* Cancer;
    Cardiovascular disease
    fitness and, 6-7, 10
    screening for risk for, 12-13
    smoking and, 6, 7, 62, 81-82
Diuretic fluids, 64
Diverticulosis, 7
Dragging, skill level required
    for, 5
Dropping out, 103, 104-106
Drug abuse. *See* Alcohol abuse;
    Substance abuse
Duration of exercise. *See* Time
    for exercise

E

Early retirement, 9
Eating log, 66, 67, 72
Emphysema, 7, 81, 82
Endurance. *See* Cardiovascular
    endurance; Muscular
    strength and endurance
Energy balance, 69-70
Environmental guidelines for
    training, 34-36
Excessive force, 9
Exercise. *See also* Fitness pro-
    gram design; Principles of
    exercise
    smoking and, 83
    stress and, 77
    for weight management, 71,
        72
Exercise machine exercises, 42,
    43
Expectations, realistic, 107. *See
    also* Goal setting

F

Fagerstrom Tolerance Test, 83,
    84
Fat, body. *See* Body composition
Fats, nutritional, 7, 62-63, 66
Fiber intake, 7, 66
Fitness. *See also* Fitness level sta-
    tistics
    causes of lack of, 8
    components defined, 4-5
    definition of, 3
    importance to law enforce-
        ment, 5-6

Fitness contracts, 108, 109
Fitness level statistics
    for Americans in general, 6-7
    for law enforcement officers,
        8-9
Fitness profiling, 97-98
Fitness program benefits, 9-10
Fitness program design
    for anaerobic fitness, 56-58
    for calisthenics, 45-47
    for cardiovascular
        endurance, 30-36
    for flexibility, 50-54
    general exercise principles
        for, 23-27
    for muscular strength and
        endurance, 39-47
    for resistance training, 38, 39-
        45
    for weight management, 70-
        73
Fitness testing, 11-20
    by agencies, 13
    body composition assess-
        ment, 71-72
    for progress checks, 96-97
    screening before, 11-13
    self-testing, 13-20
        instructions for test items,
            14-18
        interpreting results of, 18
        Screening Tests for, 13-14
FITT formula. *See also*
    Frequency of exercise;
    Intensity of exercise; Time
    for exercise; Type of exer-
    cise, definition of
    for anaerobic fitness training,
        56-57, 58
    for cardiovascular endurance
        training, 31-32, 36
    definition of, 27
    for flexibility training, 50-51,
        54
    for resistance training, 39-40,
        42, 46
Flexed-arm hangs (exercise), 46
Flexibility, 49-54. *See also*
    Stretching
    benefits of, 10, 50
    current levels among officers,
        8
    definition of, 5, 49-50

fitness test for, 16
law enforcement requirements for, 50
physiological processes for, 49-50
training program for, 50-54
Fluids, 64
Force, use of, 5, 9
Free weight exercises, 42, 43, 44-45, 111-114
Frequency of exercise. *See also* FITT formula
for anaerobic fitness training, 58
for cardiovascular endurance training, 36
definition of, 27
for flexibility training, 54
for resistance training, 42, 46
Full range of motion (FROM)
for flexibility training, 53
for resistance training, 44

G

Gallbladder disease, 7
Gender, and resistance training, 38
Goal setting, 95-102
benefits of, 95
examples of, 98-101
general considerations for, 95-96
how to set specific goals, 97-98, 101-102
progress evaluation and, 96-97
worksheet for, 101-102
Groin stretch (exercise), 117
Group training, motivational advantages of, 107

H

Half-knee bends (exercise), 43, 46, 111-112
Hamstrings stretch (exercise), 116
HDL (high-density lipoprotein), 63
Health. *See also* Disease
alcohol abuse and, 7, 89
body composition and, 70

fitness and, 6-7, 9, 10
nutrition and, 62-63, 66, 67
smoking and, 6, 7, 62, 81-83
stress and, 7, 8, 76-77
Health care costs, 6, 7, 10, 81
Health history screening. *See* Screening
Heart disease. *See* Cardiovascular disease
Heart rate
for cardiovascular endurance training, 31-32
instructions for measuring, 14
Heart rate reserve (HRR), 31
Heel raises (exercise), 43, 46, 111
High altitude, and training, 34-35
High blood pressure (hypertension)
causes of, 7, 66, 70, 76
consequences of, 82
statistics on, 6
High-density lipoprotein (HDL), 63
Hip flexor stretch (exercise), 117
Hot weather, training in, 34, 35
HRR (heart rate reserve), 31
Humid weather, training in, 34, 35
Hypertension. *See* High blood pressure
Hypothermia, 34

I

Image, professional, 5, 6, 70
Individuality principle
definition of, 23
for flexibility training, 50
Injuries
body composition and, 70
fitness and, 6, 10
nutrition and, 67
prevention during training, 27, 34-36, 43, 44, 45, 53, 54, 58
Intensity of exercise. *See also* FITT formula
for anaerobic fitness training, 56, 58
for cardiovascular endurance training, 31-32, 36

definition of, 27
for flexibility training, 50-51, 54
for resistance training, 39-40, 46
International Association of Chiefs of Police, 8, 9
Isokinetic contractions, 38
Isometric contractions, 38
Isotonic contractions, 38

J

Job performance, benefits of fitness for, 9, 10. *See also* Law enforcement activities
Job task simulation testing, 13
Journal of the American Medical Association, 83
Jumping, skill level required for, 5

K

Karvonen formula, 31-32

L

Law and Order magazine, 6, 9
Law enforcement activities
anaerobic power requirements for, 56
cardiovascular endurance requirements for, 4, 5, 30
effect of weight management on, 5, 70
flexibility requirements for, 50
general benefits of fitness for, 5-6, 9
muscular strength/endurance requirements for, 39
skill requirements summarized, 5-6
LDL (low-density lipoprotein), 62
Leg curl (exercise), 46
Leg flexion (exercise), 43, 112
Lifestyle factors. *See* Nutrition; Obesity; Sedentary living; Smoking; Smoking cessation; Stress; Substance abuse

Lifting and carrying, skill level required for, 5
Log, of food consumption, 66, 67, 72
Longevity, 10
Low-density lipoprotein (LDL), 62
Lower-back pain, 7, 15, 76
Lower back stretch (exercise), 118
Lower leg stretch (exercise), 115
Lung cancer, 6, 7, 81, 82, 83

M

Marijuana abuse, 87
Maximum heart rate (MHR), 31
Maximum oxygen uptake ($\dot{V}O_2$max), 17, 19-20
Maximum push-up test, 15, 19-20
MHR (maximum heart rate), 31
Military press (exercise), 43, 114
Minerals, 64, 65
Mode of exercise. *See* Type of exercise, definition of
Moderation principle, 27
Monounsaturated fats, 63
Mortality statistics, 6, 7, 9, 81, 82, 83
Motivation, 106-108
MSE. *See* Muscular strength and endurance
Multijurisdictional Law Enforcement Physical Skills Survey, 5
Muscle contractions, 38
Muscle fibers, 39
Muscular strength and endurance (MSE), 37-47
  benefits of, 10, 39
  body composition and, 70
  current levels among officers, 8
  definition of, 4, 37-38
  fitness test for, 15-16
  law enforcement requirements for, 39
  physiological processes for, 38-39
  training program for, 39-47

N

National Law Enforcement Fitness Test, 13
Neck stretch (exercise), 119
Nicotine patches, 83
Norms
  definition of, 97
  table of, 19-20
Nutrition, 61-67
  basic goals for, 65-67
  costs of illness and, 6
  definition of, 61
  importance of, 7
  role of specific nutrients in, 61-65
  for weight management, 66, 70-71, 72-73

O

Obesity. *See also* Weight management
  consequences of, 7
  nutrition and, 67
One and one-half mile run test, 17-18, 19-20
One-mile walk test, 16-17
One-minute sit-up test, 14, 19-20
One-repetition maximum (1RM), 39-40, 42
Organizational benefits of fitness, 10
Osteoporosis, 7
Outcome goals, 96
Overload principle
  for anaerobic fitness training, 56-57
  for cardiovascular endurance training, 31-32
  definition of, 24
  for flexibility training, 50-51
  for resistance training, 31-32
Ozone, 36

P

Pacific Life Mutual, 6
PAR-Q Preparticipation Checklist, 11-12
Partner-assisted stretching, 52
Pectoral stretch (exercise), 120
Penn State Aging Study, 8

Perceived exertion, 32, 33
Performance goals, 96
Personal inventory worksheet, 100, 101
Physical fitness. *See* Fitness
Physical fitness testing. *See* Fitness testing
Physical skills for law enforcement. *See* Law enforcement activities
Planning, and motivation, 107
Pollution, and training, 35-36
Polyunsaturated fats, 63
Positive thinking, 106
Power, aerobic. *See* Cardiovascular endurance
Power, anaerobic. *See* Anaerobic fitness/power
Practice, and motivation, 106
Preparticipation Checklist, 11-12
Prescription drug abuse, 89-90
Principles of exercise. *See also* FITT formula
  for anaerobic fitness training, 56-57
  for cardiovascular endurance training, 31-34
  definition of, 23-27
  for flexibility training, 50-53
  for resistance training, 39-40, 42-44
Productivity, 10
Professional image, 5, 6, 70
Professional organizations, 123
Programs. *See* Fitness program benefits; Fitness program design
Progress checks, 13-14, 96-97
Progression principle
  for anaerobic fitness training, 57
  for cardiovascular endurance training, 32-33
  definition of, 24
  for flexibility training, 51
  for resistance training, 42
Proteins, nutritional, 63-64
Pulse rate, instructions for measuring, 14. *See also* Heart rate
Pushing, skill level required for, 5
Push-ups (exercise)
  for fitness testing, 15, 19-20
  for resistance training, 46

Q

Quadriceps stretch (exercise), 117

R

Rating of perceived exertion (RPE), 32, 33
Raw scores, conversion of, 97
Recovery principle
  for anaerobic fitness training, 57
  for cardiovascular endurance training, 33-34
  definition of, 25-26
  for flexibility training, 52-53
  for resistance training, 42
Regularity principle
  for anaerobic fitness training, 57
  for cardiovascular endurance training, 33
  definition of, 25
  for flexibility training, 52
  for resistance training, 42
Relaxation techniques, 78
Resistance training, 38, 39-45. *See also* Free weight exercises
Resting heart rate, 14
Retirement statistics, 9
Reversibility principle, 26-27
Rewards, 107
Risk factors, screening for, 12-13
RPE (rating of perceived exertion), 32, 33
Running, skill level required for, 5

S

Salt intake, 66
Saturated fats, 63, 66
Score conversion, 97-98
Screening
  before fitness testing, 11-13
  for monitoring progress, 13-14
Screening Tests, 13-14. *See also* Screening
Sedentary living, 7

Selye, Hans, 31
Setbacks, 105-106
Shoulder stretch (exercise), 120
Sick days, 10
Sit-and-reach test, 16, 19-20
Sit-ups (exercise)
  for fitness testing, 14, 19-20
  for resistance training, 43, 46, 112
Skills. *See* Law enforcement activities
Smoking, 81-85
  consequences of, 6, 7, 62, 81-82
  guidelines for quitting, 83-84
  second-hand smoke, 7, 82-83
  statistics on, 6, 7, 81-82, 83
Smoking cessation
  guidelines for, 83-84
  success rate statistics, 81, 83
Sodium intake, 66
Specificity principle
  for anaerobic fitness training, 57
  for cardiovascular endurance training, 33
  definition of, 24-25
  for flexibility training, 51
  for resistance training, 42
Spotting, for weight training, 45
Squats (half-knee bends; exercise), 43, 46, 111-112
Stamina. *See* Cardiovascular endurance
Standard, definition of, 97
Static stretching, 52, 54, 115-121
Steroid use, 7, 87, 90
Strength. *See* Muscular strength and endurance
Stress, 75-79
  causes of, 8, 75
  consequences of, 7, 8, 76-77
  definition of, 75
  fitness for reduction of, 10
  negative ways of coping with, 8, 76, 82
  physical symptoms of, 75
  statistics on, 60, 76
  techniques for management of, 76, 77-79
  weight management and, 73
Stretching. *See also* Flexibility
  exercise instructions, 53, 115-121

types of, 51-52
  for warming up/cooling down, 14, 54
Stroke, 81, 83
Substance abuse, 87-91. *See also* Alcohol abuse
  recreational drug abuse, 87, 89-90
  steroid use, 7, 87, 90
Suicide, 9, 76
Sulfur dioxide, 36
Supervision, and motivation, 106

T

THR (training heart rate), 31
Three hundred-meter run, 57-58
Time for exercise. *See also* FITT formula
  for anaerobic fitness training, 56-57, 58
  for cardiovascular endurance training, 32, 36
  definition of, 27
  for flexibility training, 51, 54
  for resistance training, 40, 42, 46
Tobacco use. *See* Smoking; Smoking cessation
Total fitness, defined, 3. *See also* Fitness
Training heart rate (THR), 31
Training programs. *See* Fitness program benefits; Fitness program design
Triceps extension (exercise), 43, 114
Triceps stretch (exercise), 121
Trunk lifts (exercise), 43, 46, 112-113
Trunk stretch (exercise), 119
Type of exercise, definition of, 27. *See also* FITT formula

U

Unsaturated fats, 63
Upper back stretch (exercise), 119
Use of force, 5, 9

V

Variety principle
  for cardiovascular endurance
    training, 34
  definition of, 26
  for flexibility training, 53
  for resistance training, 43-44
Vitamins, 64, 65
$\dot{V}O_2$max (maximum oxygen
    uptake), 17, 19-20

W

Warm-ups
  for anaerobic fitness training,
    58
  basic guidelines, 14, 54
  for resistance training, 44
Water
  intake with hot weather
    training, 35
  in nutrition, 64
Weather conditions, and train-
    ing, 34, 35
Weight, screening test for, 14

Weight management, 69-73
  benefits of fitness for, 10
  definition of, 69
  effect on law enforcement
    activities, 5, 70
  energy balance concepts for,
    69-70
  nutrition for, 66, 70-71, 72-73
  program for, 70-73
  stress and, 73
Weight training. *See* Free weight
    exercises; Resistance train-
    ing
Wollack and Associates, 5, 6

About the Authors

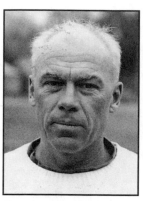

Robert Hoffman retired from the United States Army as a lieutenant colonel in 1991 and is now director of FitForce. During his 22 years in the military, Bob completed assignments around the world. He commanded a Brigade Headquarters Company in Germany, a Ranger Company in Vietnam, and a Special Forces SCUBA Detachment at Fort Bragg, NC. He also commanded the 4th Ranger Training Battalion at Fort Benning, GA, where in addition to working with Rangers, Bob trained U.S. Drug Enforcement Agents who were being deployed to South America.

Bob spent 3 years as the director of training for the army's Soldier Physical Fitness School and brought the army's fitness program into the 21st century by helping to develop the army's Total Fitness program. He also spent 4 years as a professor in the Department of Physical Education at West Point. While there, he was an assistant cross-country and track coach and a junior varsity basketball coach.

Bob holds a master's degree in physical education from Indiana University. He is certified as a fitness instructor by the American College of Sports Medicine and as a Master Fitness Trainer by the U.S. Army. He is a member of the American Society of Law Enforcement Trainers. Bob is the author of *Running Together: The Family Book of Jogging,* and he helped write the army's *Physical Fitness Training* field manual. Bob lives in Champaign, IL.

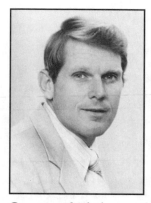

Prior to serving as the technical adviser for FitForce, **Thomas R. Collingwood** worked at the Cooper Institute for Aerobics Research in Dallas, TX, for 13 years. While there, Tom initiated the institute's involvement in law enforcement fitness and created the Police Fitness Instructors Course, which he used to train more than 7,000 police fitness instructors. He has helped more than 200 law enforcement agencies design fitness programs and standards and has also conducted more than 30 fitness standards validation studies within federal, state, and local law enforcement agencies.

Tom was a military policeman with the U.S. Army, a police psychologist for the Dallas Police Department, and training director for the Kentucky Department of Justice. He has served as the national fitness director for the American Society of Law Enforcement Trainers and as a special consultant/clinician on law enforcement fitness to the President's Council on Physical Fitness and Sports and the International Association of Chiefs of Police (IACP).

Tom holds a master's degree in exercise science from the University of Kentucky and a doctorate in psychology from the State University of New York at Buffalo. He has been recognized for his work in the field of law enforcement fitness by the IACP, the U.S. Drug Enforcement Administration, the U.S. Marshals Service, and the U.S. Secret Service. He is also the recipient of the Healthy American Fitness Leaders award presented by the President's Council on Physical Fitness and Sports and the National Jaycees. Tom resides in Dallas, TX.

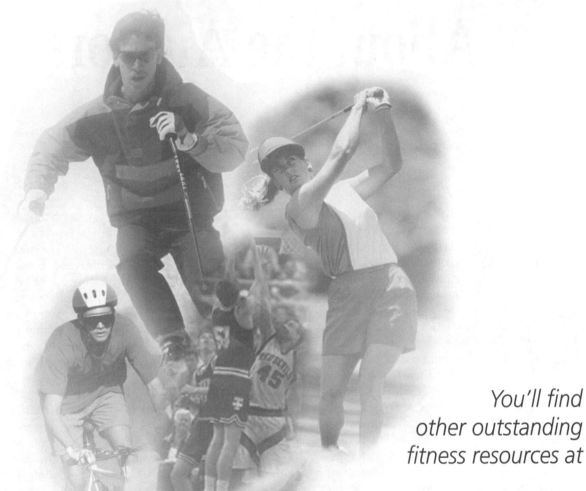